THE PRACTICE AND PROCESS

Health Education
in Health Promotion

Sheila Hill Parker

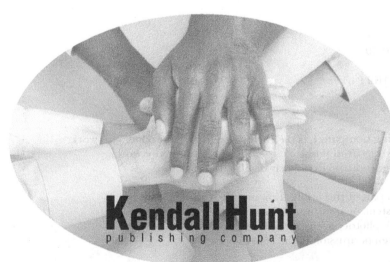

Kendall Hunt
publishing company

Cover image © Shutterstock, Inc. Used under license.

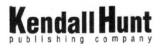

www.kendallhunt.com
Send all inquiries to:
4050 Westmark Drive
Dubuque, IA   52004-1840

Table of Contents

Appendices

community health and public health need … … health education and … … … … … … … health … Finally, the book … … … … … … … … … … … … … … … health education … … … … … … … health education and … … … … … … … … … … … … … health education … … … … … … in health promotion.

Preface

Many students come to the study of health education and health promotion because they have a personal interest in health. Yet many of these students would have difficulty defining what health is beyond their personal interests. Most have not encountered anyone whose profession is actually centered in health education and health promotion beyond their school health teacher. Due to the economic challenges that our society is facing in education, many school systems may not have formally trained school health education specialists. So many students may only have encountered teachers from other subject areas attempting to teach a health course or a few sessions in middle school or high school. Sometimes these experiences have been good learning experiences for the students and sometimes not. However, it is quite possible that these learning experiences have not opened the doors to the many opportunities for learning and experiences that exist in the health field.

As a member of the faculty in a college of public health, it is indeed exciting to observe students who for the first time begin to see and experience the meaning of health and the many professions that serve to help people improve and maintain their health locally, nationally, and globally. The students that experience this awakening are energized by the many opportunities that exist for careers in public health and community health in which they can actually help people change and enhance the quality of their lives. They learn that through health education and health promotion they can gain knowledge and skills that can bring important changes to the lives of individuals and communities.

This book is written to introduce students to the meaning of health and its role in the lives of individuals, communities, and nations. Students will learn the historical context for health and the rise of the professions in health education and health promotion. The book takes the student from observing actual health concerns of a family and its members to the profession that is designed to address these concerns. The student is introduced to the purpose, the roles and the responsibilities of the health education profession. The book approaches health education as one of the important core professions in health promotion. Most importantly, the book introduces students in

v

community health and public health majors to the health education process that has contributed greatly to the work of changing health behaviors for improved quality of life through research, theory, and evidence-based interventions and programming. Finally the book is designed to accompany instructors' skill-building activities in using the health education process for program planning in health education and health promotion.

Prologue

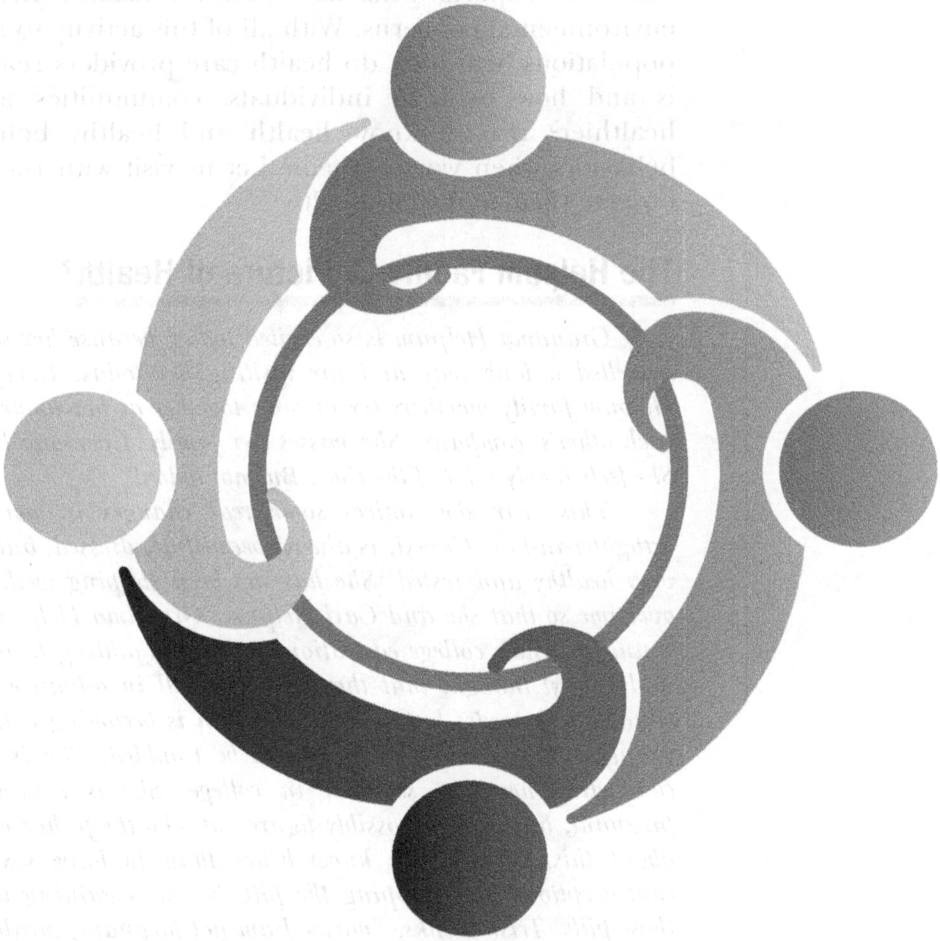

As students of public health or community health, you are most likely planning for a career in the health care field. Many of you may hope to make major contributions to making populations at home or abroad healthier with improved opportunities to live healthier and happier lives. Have you considered how you will accomplish this goal?

There is much discussion currently about health. Many people are searching for the answers to their personal health challenges and problems. Many who are healthy are seeking ways to prolong their present health or to enhance it. Researchers are dedicated to discovering the answers to the many health problems that nations and the world face daily through medicine, lifestyle changes, social changes, and environmental changes. Governmental agencies produce guidelines on what the experts consider optimum healthy lifestyle behaviors and environmental concerns. With all of this activity to make individuals and populations healthier, do health care providers really know what health is and how to help individuals, communities and nations become healthier? Do we know health and healthy behaviors or unhealthy behaviors when we see them? Let us visit with the Helpum family and observe them and their health.

The Helpum Family: A Picture of Health?

Grandma Helpum is so excited today, because her son and his family have travelled a long way and are visiting her today. Every two years, all of the Helpum family members try to come together at her home to reminisce and enjoy each other's' company. She misses her family. Everyone has moved so far away. She feels lonely a lot of the time. But not today!

This year she notices some real changes in her family members. Her daughter-in-law, Cheryl, is always beautifully dressed, but today she does not look very healthy and rested. She has not been sleeping well. She has been working overtime so that she and Carl Helpum, Grandma Helpum's son, can pay for the youngest child's college education and avoid adding to their growing debt. Carl and Cheryl thought that they planned well in advance to meet their children's educational needs, but college education is becoming extremely expensive. Their youngest daughter, Trish, seems to be troubled. She is 18 years old and just completing her first semester in college. She is concerned that she may be pregnant, but cannot possibly figure out who the father might be. She feels badly about this, because she knew better than to have sex without some sort of contraception after stopping the pill. She was gaining too much weight taking those pills. Trish thinks, "maybe I am not pregnant, maybe I am just getting fat." She wonders what this will do to her parents if she is pregnant; they work so hard to give her a great education and everything that she wants. Well, at least she is not having problems like her brother, Michael, who is supposed to be building his career in the banking industry. However, he seems to be spending a lot of money on his fancy car and seems high all of the time. He always has an entourage of young women following him, most of whom he does not know. Carl Helpum is suspicious about what his son might be doing. He intends to have a long talk with him, but Carl cannot seem to find the time to talk to Michael, because Carl is always busy; always working to stay ahead of the younger men and women in his organization who are frequently trying to take his position. He finds himself smoking more and drinking alcohol more than ever before.

Here comes Grandma Helpum with her camera. "Let's take pictures! I want all of my friends to see my beautiful and healthy family!"

Chapter 1

Health Defined, Health Dimensions and Health Determinants

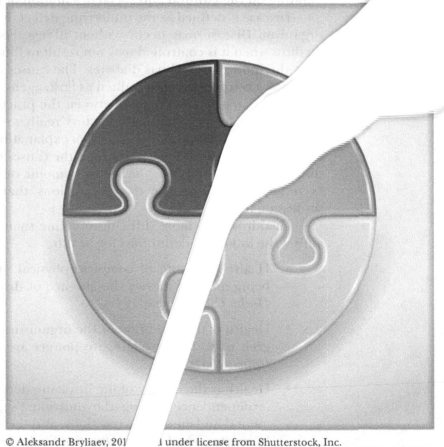

Health Defined

Health professionals and those preparing to be health professionals in health education and health promotion seek to understand health and to improve it for the populations and individuals that they serve. There can be no successful efforts to improve health without a clear understanding of what health is. In their efforts, health professionals will realize that people may ascribe definitions for health, illness, and disease that are not the same across populations and cultures.

For many generations, health was defined as the absence of illness and disease. Unlike the definition for health, the definitions for illness and disease may seem fairly straightforward. Illness is defined as the visible presentation of symptoms which make one feel distressed. Illness can be observed objectively by the health professional. However, for the lay person illness may mean being sick and in need of help from someone who can provide relief. The person providing relief may be a physician, folk healer, or other practitioner identified formally or informally, depending on the cultural and social orientation of the sick person.

Disease is defined as the underlying defect or malfunction within the organism. Disease may occur without illness. For an example, diabetes mellitus when it is controlled may not result in illness from diabetes. However, the individual still has diabetes. The causes of diseases and illnesses are often explored and determined as host, agent, and environmental factors. There may be differences between the practitioner and the population in determining what these factors really are. The sociocultural aspects of illness and disease present other explanations, besides carcinogens, bacteria, viruses, etc., for determining the causes or agents for illness and disease, such as "soul loss," "evil eye," demonic or spirit possession, spells, even another person for the populations that are served by health professionals.

Health is even more difficult to define than illness and disease. Examine the following definitions for health.

- Health is a state of complete physical, mental, and social well-being and not merely the absence of disease or infirmity *(World Health Organization, 1947)*.

- Health is the condition of the organism, which measures the degree to which its aggregate powers are able to function *(Oberteuffer, 1965)*.

- Health is the quality of life involving dynamic interaction and interdependence among the individual's physical well-being, his mental and emotional reactions, and the social complex in which he exists *(School Health Education Study, 1967)*.

- An integrated method of functioning which is oriented toward maximizing the potential of which the individual is capable. It requires that the individual maintain a continuum of balance and purposeful direction with the environment where he is functioning *(Dunn, 1967)*.

- Health is a state of being—a quality of life. It is something that defies definition in any precise, measurable sense. It is affected by a host of physical, mental, social, and spiritual factors which no single profession or academic discipline can effectively monitor and study *(Greene and Simons-Morton, 1990)*.

Examining these definitions, illustrates that health can be so many things, because it truly does affect so many aspects of life and is in turn affected by a great many factors. These are not likely to be the ways that the lay constituency would define health. One important factor that is observed by many health practitioners and lay persons is that health is not static, it is dynamic. The individual is always required to adapt to various factors that can impact his or her health positively or negatively. One moment an individual may be healthy, but in another instance may become ill. Health and illness cannot coexist. However, those who suffer from a disease, but who are effectively managing the disease may actually experience a high level of health.

Perhaps the following definition can best serve as a general definition that works for the professional and the populations that are served by the professionals.

Health is the combination of the physical, psychological, social, and spiritual dimensions of life that can be balanced in a way that produces satisfaction and joy in life.

The definition implies that humans are not one dimensional, but multidimensional. They are not static, but dynamic, constantly impacting or being impacted by their environments. The concept of balance in these dimensions of health implies that one can compensate for the lower level of health in one dimension by improving the levels of other dimensions of health. The definition implies that the balance of these dimensions will result in satisfaction that brings a sense of fulfillment and joy that is evoked by well-being and success as the individual lives a full and healthy life. The joy that is produced is more than momentary happiness; joy is both the result of and the perpetuation of hope, faith, and love (Nobles, 2010). Healthy people are joyful people who can weather the storms and the sunshine of life's circumstances and conditions. Health, then, if viewed holistically, will impact every aspect of one's life and also be impacted by many factors in life, within the physical, social, cultural, and political environments that surround every individual. Health is not an end in itself, but the means to an end or the life goals of the individual or population.

So what exactly are these dimensions of health and what do they involve?

Dimensions of Health

Figure 1.1 Dimensions of Health

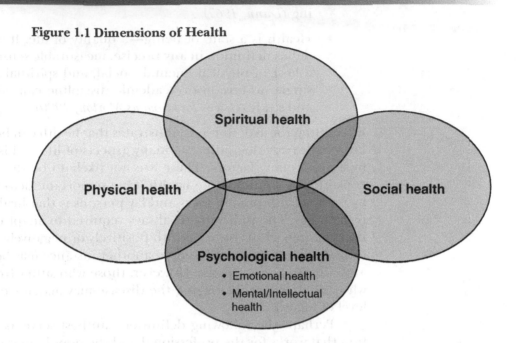

The origin of the word "health" is derived from the Old English word "*hale*," meaning wholeness, being whole, sound or well, strong, uninjured, of good omen—cognate with holy and implies involvement of the entire individual. Clearly this means more than the physical dimension. The nature and number of dimensions which comprise health have been debated, but health researchers and professionals are in agreement that there are varying dimensions of health and that these dimensions function in an integrated, coordinated way, never in isolation, to produce health in the individual (Dolfman, 1973). For the purposes of this text, the author presents four primary dimensions of health that can be balanced to produce joy and satisfaction:

- Physical Health
- Psychological Health (Emotional Health, Mental/Intellectual Health)
- Social Health
- Spiritual Health

Physical Health

Physical health is defined as the absence of disease and disability. It implies that the individual is functioning adequately from the perspective of physical and physiological abilities. Physical health relates to the biological integrity of the individual, incorporating the following:

- body size and shape
- sensory acuity
- susceptibility to disease
- body functioning and recuperative ability

Psychological Health

Psychological health is the appropriate intellectual, mental, and emotional practices and dimensions of the individual. Generally, psychological health reflects the following:

- values and belief systems as well as our level of self-esteem, and self-confidence
- coping skills and mechanisms
- hardiness

Within psychological health, the emotional health aspect is generally defined as the ability to feel and express the full range of human emotions, giving and receiving love, achieving a sense of fulfillment and purpose in life, and developing psychological hardiness. Mental or intellectual health encompasses the intellectual processes of reasoning, analysis, evaluation, curiosity, humor, alertness, logic, learning, and memory.

Social Health

Social health refers to the ability to perform and fulfill the expectations of our roles in society, "effectively, comfortably, with pleasure, without harming other people" (Butler, 2001). An individual's social health includes, but is not limited to the following:

- interactions and connections with others
- the ability to adapt to various social situations
- the daily behaviors and actions
- the ability to communicate effectively
- the ability to show respect
- a sense of belonging within a larger social context
- having responsibilities that often affect others and involve meeting their needs
- needs for love, intimacy, companionship, safety, and cooperation

Spiritual Health

Spiritual health has been defined by Hawks (1994) as "a high level of faith, hope, and commitment in relation to a well-defined worldview or belief system that provides a sense of meaning and purpose to existence, and that offers an ethical path to personal fulfillment which includes connectedness with self, others, and a higher power or larger reality." Banks (1980) and Butler (2001) find that the spiritual dimension of health has a unifying force within the individual that integrates all of the other dimensions of health, affecting the total health and well-being. Spiritual health may or may not be reflected in religious practices. Spiritual health is the core that makes the following possible:

- the ability to discover, articulate, and act on one's basic purpose in life,

- learning how to give and receive love, joy, and peace,

- contributing to the improvement of the spiritual health of others,

- pursuing a fulfilling and meaningful life,

- transcending the self with a sense of selflessness, or empathy, for others and establishing a commitment to a power beyond the natural and rational,

- having the power to pursue successes in life through a defined set of moral principles and ethics.

Some research indicates that the spiritual component may actually provide the unifying context for all other components of health.

Other Health-Related Definitions

Wellness

While the terms "health" and "wellness" are often used interchangeably, they are not synonyms (Penhollow, 2012). Wellness is a concept that describes the process of adopting behaviors that determine one's quality of life. Anspaugh et. al., (1997) pronounced that wellness means engaging in attitudes and behaviors that enhance the quality of life and maximize personal potential. The dimensions of wellness are very similar to those in the description of health, but may also include the dimensions of environmental, and occupational wellness. Often health professionals refer to the wellness scale that indicates the quality of life as a range from optimal wellness to premature death. The individual can choose to exercise control over a variety of life factors that will influence the level or ranking of wellness. The more positive life factors present in a person's life at any given time, the greater is the likelihood of optimal health and wellness. If one approaches wellness as a continuum with the midpoint as no signs or symptoms of disease, as in Figure 1.2, one's choices in behaviors can move the individual toward illness or premature death or the individual may choose behaviors that move him/her toward wellness and optimal health.

Figure 1.2 A Continuum for Wellness

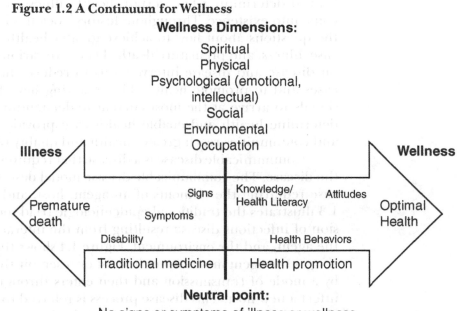

Wellness Dimensions:
Spiritual
Physical
Psychological (emotional, intellectual)
Social
Environmental
Occupation

Illness — **Wellness**

Premature death — Optimal Health

Signs — Knowledge/Health Literacy — Attitudes
Symptoms
Disability — Health Behaviors
Traditional medicine — Health promotion

Neutral point:
No signs or symptoms of illness or wellness

Personal Health

Personal health is the actions and decisions made by the individual that affect his or her own health. It is important to note that some of the decisions and actions may be impacted by factors outside of the person's control.

Community Health and Population Health

People interact with each other in many ways for many reasons. We commonly refer to these interactions with common bonds as community. Community is defined as a unified body of people with common interests living in a particular area; an interacting population of various kinds of individuals in a common location; or, a "body of persons with a common history, ethnic heritage, political interests, or social and economic characteristics (Merriam-Webster Dictionary, 2013). Community health refers to the health status, issues, activities, and events of a community. This includes the organized responsibilities of public health, school health, transportation safety, other tax-supported functions, with voluntary and private actions, to promote and protect the health of local populations identified as communities. Sometimes the term population health is used. Population health refers to the health status and the conditions influencing the health of a category of people (for example, women, adolescents, prisoners) whether or not the people included in the category define themselves as a community.

Determinants of Health

An examination of the health of individuals and communities will lead to determining how certain health, illness, and disease conditions come into existence. Throughout history, societies have sought answers to the questions about how to achieve greater health and avoid injury, disease, illness, and premature death. There are various models and theories on disease and disease interventions to reduce the transmission of diseases and to promote health. The following have helped health professionals to arrive at the most current understandings about what factors determine health and enable health care providers to help individuals and communities reach greater health and quality of their lives.

Communicable disease is a disease that requires a pathogen to spread the disease. The communicable disease model describes the spread of disease requiring the elements of an agent, host, and environment. Figure 1.3 illustrates the traditional epidemiologic triad model for the transmission of infectious disease resulting from the interaction among the host, the agent, and the environment. Figure 1.4 shows the transmission occurring as the agent moves from the host or reservoir through a portal of exit by a mode of transmission and then enters through a portal of entry to infect a new host. This disease process is referred to as the chain of infection and will continue until the chain is broken.

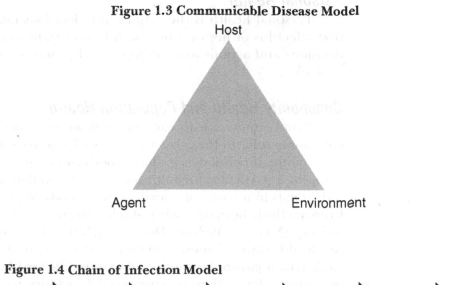

Figure 1.3 Communicable Disease Model

Figure 1.4 Chain of Infection Model

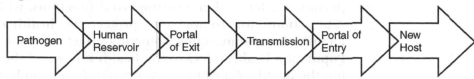

These models do help the health professionals working in health education and health promotion explain and intervene in reducing the spread of communicable or infectious disease. In more recent years, there is greater knowledge and experience related to diseases that are communicable and those that are the result of lifestyle choices. Canada in the 1970's implemented a national plan to insure health care for all Canadians. Canadian health professionals began to examine the health field rather than the health care system to broaden their assessment of the many matters that impact and affect the health of their people. The Lalonde Report, *A New Perspective on the Health of Canadians* (1974), introduced the concept of the "health field" which at that time consisted of four categories of elements that could influence death and disease for humans: human biology or heredity, environment, lifestyle or behavior, and inadequacies of the health care services. Shortly after the Lalonde Report the United States government officially entered health promotion with the publication of *Healthy People: The Surgeon General's Report on Health Promotion and Disease Prevention* (1979). No longer was the focus totally on the treatment of disease, but the emphasis moved to the prevention of illness and health promotion.

For many years, the Health Field Concept provided a framework that is used by many health professionals to identify causes of morbidity and mortality, by examining the contributions of heredity, environment, health care services, and behavior to a variety of health conditions and problems. In the most recent years, the Health Field Concept has yielded to the use of the term "determinants of health," as a way to assess and explain the many factors that determine the health of populations. According to McGinnis, et. al., (2001), the impacts of these determinants on premature mortality are distributed as ". . . genetic predispositions, about 30%, social circumstances, 15%, environmental exposures, 5%, behavioral patterns, 40%; and shortfalls in medical care about 10%." It is important to note that while these determinants are listed individually, they do interact and interconnect having impacts on each other and reflecting the total health of the individual, the family, and the community.

According to the 2011 Joint Committee on Health Education and Health Promotion Terminology (2012), determinants of health are "the range of personal, social, economic, and environmental factors that influence health status." The categories of determinants affecting individual and community levels of health are:

- Genetic Factors/ Heredity (Micro/Internal Environment)
- Physical Environment
- Social Environment
- Health Care
- Personal Health Behavior And Lifestyle Choices

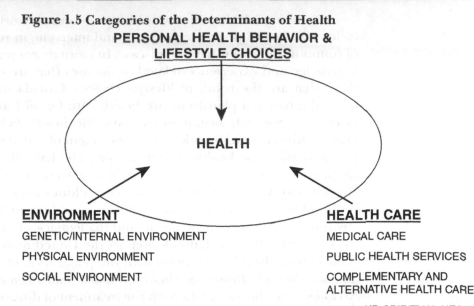

Figure 1.5 Categories of the Determinants of Health

**PERSONAL HEALTH BEHAVIOR &
LIFESTYLE CHOICES**

HEALTH

ENVIRONMENT

GENETIC/INTERNAL ENVIRONMENT

PHYSICAL ENVIRONMENT

SOCIAL ENVIRONMENT

HEALTH CARE

MEDICAL CARE

PUBLIC HEALTH SERVICES

COMPLEMENTARY AND
ALTERNATIVE HEALTH CARE

FOLK AND SPIRITUAL HEALING

Genetic Factors/Heredity

Generally, it is believed that there are a number of factors affecting our health over which we have little control. However, it may be difficult to separate the influences of heredity from those of culture and social circumstances for individuals and groups of people. The genetic factors determining the health of individuals and populations include the following:

- Genetic traits affecting optimal functioning
- Sex
- Body size and composition

The Physical Environment

The physical environment has great importance and influence on the health of individuals and communities. Increasingly, individuals, communities, and health professionals understand how pollution and contamination of the water, air, and food supply are linked to greater incidence and prevalence of a variety of diseases and allergic reactions. Some of the determinants of health in the physical environment are:

- Air
- Water
- Soil

- Animal life
- Plant life
- Natural disasters

The Social Environment

Social scientists and social epidemiologists examine the relationships of health problems and social factors. They try to determine the influence on health and their associations with health. Research has documented the importance of social variables in predicting and describing health and health problems. John Ratcliffe (1980) believed that society's social structure greatly affects the lives and the health of all people.

In many communities, socially designed systems have become more important than the physical environment to individual survival, because they control the distribution of and access to those very factors that determine mortality and morbidity levels. To be sure, the physical environment still exacts a great toll through incidents such as hurricanes, tornadoes, earthquakes, tidal waves, floods, etc. Nevertheless, the socioeconomic systems created by and for people constitute, to all intents and purposes, the human individual's "natural" environment (Ratcliffe, 1980). Some of the following factors can determine the health and quality of life for individuals and populations.

- Culture
- Socioeconomic factors
  - Social class
  - Personal income
  - Economy
  - Residence
- Politics
- Race and ethnicity
- Education
- Gender
- Religion
- Resources
- Community & societal organization
- Population density
- Crowding
- The pace of modern civilization

- Stressful life events
- War
- The health care environment

Health Care

Access to quality medical care and public health services can help individuals and populations experience better health. However, health care professionals must always be conscious that diverse populations may also participate in complementary and alternative health care, as well as folk healing and spiritual healing experiences. The determinants of health care will include the following:

- Medical care
- Public health services
- Complementary and alternative health care
- Folk and spiritual healing

Personal Health Behaviors and Lifestyle Choices

Most advances in optimal health and wellness in the United States have not resulted from advances in medical care, but from many of the environmental improvements and public health advances. Evidence demonstrates that the most important factors in improving health in modern societies have been improved nutrition, well-nourished babies, children, and adolescents, and relative affluence. The individual can make lifestyle changes that affect health positively or negatively, in spite of the social environment. It is in this category of determinants that health educators focus great effort. Behavior changes have great impact on health and the quality of one's life. The leading causes of death in the United States are cancers and cardiovascular diseases, which are strongly linked to lifestyle and behaviors. The following factors are supported by much research and have greatly impacted on improved health.

- Nutritional and dietary behaviors and status
- Physical activity and exercise patterns
- Adequate sleep
- Maintaining appropriate weight
- Avoidance of inappropriate use of alcohol and illegal drugs
- No tobacco use

- Prevention of unintentional injuries
- Appropriate management of stress
- Use of preventive health services

Just as there are behaviors that support optimal health there are also behaviors that cause health problems (Kolbe, 1993).

- Drug and alcohol abuse
- Risky behaviors that result in unintentional and intentional injuries
- Sexual behaviors that result in unwanted pregnancy and sexually transmitted diseases, including HIV infection
- Tobacco use
- Excessive consumption of fat and calories
- Insufficient physical activity

Risk Factors

The Health Field Concept and the Determinants of Health provide those who research and practice health education and health promotion with a framework to study and intervene with health. Such a framework helps health professionals to target factors that generate or influence the health and quality of life for the individuals, groups, and communities served. The study of determinants of health assists health professionals target risks that are associated with disease or poor health outcomes. Risk factors are defined by the World Health the Organization as ". . . any attribute, characteristic or exposure of an individual that increases the likelihood of developing a disease or injury. Some examples of the more important risk factors are underweight, morbid obesity, unsafe sex, high blood pressure, tobacco and alcohol consumption, and unsafe water, sanitation and hygiene (2013)." A risk factor increases the probability of developing disease, disability, injury, or premature death, but does not guarantee that those with the risk factor will suffer poor health outcomes. Risk factors may be categorized as modifiable risk factors (changeable or controllable) or nonmodifiable risk factors (nonchangeable or noncontrollable). Modifiable risk factors may include smoking behaviors, sedentary lifestyle, poor nutritional habits, and poor dental care. Nonmodifiable risk factors are inherited genetic factors, race, age, sex: things that cannot be changed by the individual. Professionals involved in health education and health promotion have major responsibility for helping clients identify and control risk factors that are modifiable (Cottrell et. al., 2012).

Application Opportunity

Now that you have studied the definitions for health, its dimensions, and its determinants, return to your definition for health that you wrote in the prologue.

1. Is your definition, written in the prologue, the same as the definition(s) you studied in chapter 1?

2. What are the similarities?

3. What are the differences?

4. Which definition would serve you best as a health professional? Why?

References

Anspaugh, D. J., and G. Ezell. 1995. *Teaching Today's Health,* 4th ed. Boston: Allyn & Bacon.

Butler, J. Thomas. 2001. *Principles of Health Education & Health Promotion,* 3rd ed. Belmont, CA: Wadsworth/Thomason Learning.

Cottrell, R. R., J. T. Girvan, and J. F. McKenzie. 2012. *Principles and Foundations of Health Promotion and Education.* Boston: Benjamin Cummings.

Dolfman, M. L. 1973. "The Concept of Health: An Historic and Analytic Examination." *Journal of School Health* 43 (8): 491–7.

Dunn, H. 1967. *High Level Wellness.* Arlington, VA: R. W. Beatty.

Hawks, S. 1994. "Spiritual Health: Definition and Theory." *Wellness Perspectives: Research, Theory and Practice* 10 (4): 3–13.

Joint Committee on Health Education and Promotion Terminology. 2012. "Report of the 2011 Joint Committee on Health Education and Promotion Terminology." *American Journal of Health Education* 43 (2).

Kolbe, L. J. 1993. "Developing a Plan of Action to Institutionalize Comprehensive School Health Education Programs in the United States." *Journal of School Health* 63 (1): 12–13.

Laframboise, H. L. 1973. "Health Policy: Breaking It Down into Manageable Segments." *Journal of the Canadian Medical Association, 108* (February 3). 388–393.

Lalonde, M. 1974. *A New Perspective on the Health of Canadians: A Working Document.* Ottawa, Canada: Ministry of National Health and Welfare.

McGinnis, J. M., and W. H. Foege. 1993. "Actual Causes of Death in the United States." *Journal of the American Medical Association* 2 (18): 2207–12.

McGinnis, J. M., W. H. Williams-Russo, and J. R. Knickman. 2002. "The Case for More Active Policy Attention to Health Promotion." *Health Affairs* 21 (2): 78–93.

Nobles, Sherman. 2010. "Joy is Not Happiness?" *Theologia.* Retrieved May 18, 2013, from http://theologica.ning.com/profiles/blogs/joy-is-not-happiness.

Oberteuffer, D. 1960. *School Health Education: A Textbook for Teachers, Nurses, and Other Professional Personnel.* New York: Harper and Brothers.

Penhollow, T. M. 2012. *Points to Health: Theory and Practice of Health Education and Health Behavior.* Dubuque, IA: Kendall Hunt Publishing Company.

Simons-Morton, B. G., W. H. Greene, and N. Gottlieb. 1995. *Introduction to Health Education and Health Promotion.* Long Grove, IL: Waveland Press, Inc.

Sliepcevich, E. M. 1967. "Health Education: A Conceptual Approach to Curriculum Design." In E. M. Sliepcevich. *School Health Education Study*. St Paul: 3M Education Press.

World Health Organization. 1947. Preamble to the Constitution of the World Health Organization as adopted by the International Health Conference, New York, 19–22 June 1946; signed on 22 July 1946 by the representatives of 61 States (Official Records of the World Health Organization, no. 2, p. 100) and entered into force on 7 April 1948.

World Health Organization. 2013. http://www.who.int/topics/risk _factors/en/. Retrieved May 25, 2013.

Chapter 2

Health Behavior, Health Education, and Health Promotion

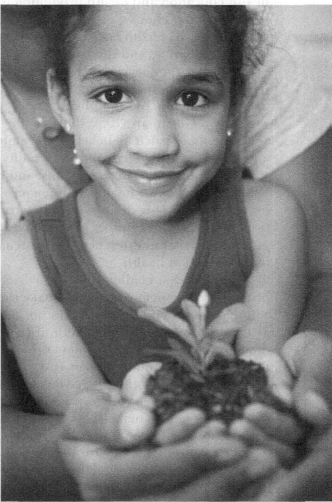

Health Behavior

While heredity, environment, and medical care have profound influences on the health and quality of life that every individual experiences, health behavior, or lifestyle is the greatest determinant that impacts morbidity and premature death. Poor health behaviors account for as much as 40% of the morbidity and premature death in the United States' population (McGinnis et. al., 2002). Lifestyle reflects practices and behavioral patterns in the individual and population that are influenced by one's cultural heritage, social relationships, social and economic circumstances, geography, and personality. While all of these factors do influence behaviors, the individual makes many decisions on his or her own, which, in turn, impact the person's health and the quality of life. Individuals can make the decision to adopt behaviors that are health enhancing or disease producing. The individual can choose to improve the level of physical activity, avoid the use of tobacco, improve the intakes of fruits and vegetables, or avoid risky sexual behavior. The foundational basis for health education and health promotion is that individuals can voluntarily make personal choices to experience the best health outcomes. It is incumbent on the health education specialists to know the factors that influence the behaviors and lifestyle choices of the individuals and target populations that they serve. Such knowledge and experience will assist the health education specialist in facilitating changed health behaviors in the target population and in individuals.

David Gochman (1982, 1997) defines health behavior as "those personal attributes such as beliefs, expectations, motive, values, perceptions and other cognitive elements; personality characteristics, including affective and emotional states and traits; and behavioral patterns, actions and habits that relate to health maintenance, health restoration, and health improvement." This definition underscores three foci for health education specialists in helping to enhance health behaviors in individuals, groups and communities: health maintenance, health restoration, and the improvement of health.

The greatest challenge to specialists in health education and health promotion is to help individuals make the best choices for health. People will make poor choices if they do not relate health to their personal life goals, if they do not value health, if they like risk-taking, and if they are unaware of the risks for sickness or death connected to their behaviors. People will make poor choices if they lack the knowledge and the skills necessary to change their behaviors to support optimal health.

There are three categories of factors that influence all of the health choices that people make. They are predisposing factors, enabling factors, and reinforcing factors.

Predisposing factors are the antecedents of a behavior; they are the things that the individual brings to the point of making a decision or choice. These factors include demographic variables such as age, sex, gender, education, race, ethnicity, and socioeconomic conditions.

Predisposing factors also consist of life experiences, values, beliefs, cultural perspectives, attitudes, and knowledge. The knowledge and attitudes may be accurate or erroneous. The health education specialists must determine what the person brings to the decision making process. This is an important key to the health education and health promotion process.

The second category of factors that influence all behaviors is enabling factors. Enabling factors are also present before the behavior occurs. Enabling factors are the person's arsenal of skills and abilities that they bring to their decisions related to behavior. Enabling factors will include the availability of health resources, affordable health care and services, or the easy availability of those things that may negatively affect health choices as well.

Reinforcing factors are the third category of factors which occur after the behavior. These are the things that can encourage the repetition of a new behavior or the extinguishing of the behavior. Reinforcing factors may include support of family and friends, feedback, and reward from instructors or employers. Often the good feelings that one experiences from improving health by a positive behavior change may help the individual to repeat the behavior, allowing the behavior to become a positive health habit.

Health Education

According to the Joint Committee on Health Education and Health Promotion Terminology (2012), health education is "Any combination of planned learning experiences using evidence based practices and/or sound theories that provide the opportunity to acquire knowledge, attitudes, and skills needed to adopt and maintain healthy behaviors." Health education is also described as a planned process that combines various educational experiences to facilitate voluntary adaptations or establishment of behaviors that are conducive to health (Green and Kreuter, 1999). The practice of health education focuses on a goal of helping people (individuals, families, groups, and communities) choose a pattern of behaviors which moves them toward optimal health rather than the reverse and to give them the ability to avoid many of the imbalances, diseases, and accidents of life (Oberteuffer et. al., 1972). Even though the field of health education has many practitioners, this goal generally describes the mission of the field and its professionals.

The fundamental principle of health education is that individuals, families, and communities can be taught to assume responsibility for their own health and, to some extent, for the health of others. The facilitation of voluntary individual and community behavior change without violating individual freedoms guaranteed by the United States Constitution is the challenge for health education professionals.

In order to bring about the voluntary changes in these persons for behaviors that support health, there is the process of health education.

Butler (2001) describes the process of health education as going beyond the memorization of information, but must also include the following:

1. The process begins with a planned intervention based on a health issue, with stated goals, objectives, activities, and evaluation criteria.

2. The intervention occurs in a specified setting and at a specified time.

3. The components of a health education intervention or program are the sequential introduction of health concepts at appropriate learning levels at each stage of the learning process and resulting in changed behaviors to support optimal health.

4. The planned intervention comprehensively helps the learner to realize how various aspects of health are interrelated and how all health behavior affects the quality of life.

5. The learner interacts with a qualified and competent educator.

In most cases the health education process improves the health knowledge base, but more importantly, there will be enriched attitudes to support behavior change, enhanced skill development, values awareness that can advance decision-making in the individual, family, and community, leading to improved health and quality of life. Positive outcomes will depend on how effectively the health education specialist plans the process.

Common misconceptions about health education are that anyone can teach health, that anyone can write an effective health education curriculum, and that health education is hygiene class. It is important to note that improving the quality of life and health status of individuals, groups, and communities are very complex and not changed in short periods of time. In examining the process for health education, the health educators must be competent in program planning, implementation, program evaluation, and in quality service delivery. Health education interventions require the health education specialist to be professionally prepared to perform various roles depending on the nature and needs of the learners. Most health education interventions will center on teaching, training counseling and consulting (Simons-Morton et. al., 1995).

Teaching

The health education specialist employs a variety of strategies, methods, and activities to help individuals, groups, and communities establish and change patterns of behavior to improve health. The health education specialist's success is dependent on what to teach and how to teach it. Conveying information alone is not sufficient to effect behavior change, because knowledge does not necessarily change attitudes or behavior.

Training

The health education specialist teaches other health professionals and volunteers how to accomplish health education goals and objectives and how to employ health education methods.

Counseling

In counseling, the health education specialist is involved in an interpersonal process of guidance that helps people learn how to achieve personal growth, improve interpersonal growth and relationships, resolve problems, make decisions, and change behavior for optimal health.

Consulting

The health education specialist employs the process by which his/her knowledge and experience are used to help another professional or organization make better decisions or cope with problems more effectively to address a group or population's health status.

The discipline and practice of health education are supported by contributions from a vast body of research in the health sciences and the social sciences that can help to reduce the risks for poor health through behavior change. The primary contributors are public health, behavioral sciences, and education. Public health contributes health statistics for epidemiologic data as the health education specialist assesses the health status of target populations. Public health also contributes to the understanding of health issues in the environment, personal lifestyles, medical care, population dynamics, biomedical science, and epidemiology. Behavioral sciences are the integration of knowledge from psychology, sociology, and cultural anthropology, providing a foundation for understanding human health behaviors. The behavioral sciences contribute greatly to defining the determinants of behavior that are key to healthful behavior change, which is the desired outcome for health education practice. Education is the study of teaching and learning which is central to health education. Education provides the health education specialist with learning theory, educational psychology, human development, curriculum development, and pedagogy. Measurement and testing are also contributions from education (Butler, 2001).

Health education has transitioned from its earliest appearance as a profession. Health education specialists are now central to the health promotion efforts that many local, state and national organizations are engaged in as these agencies seek to address the many health challenges facing the nation and the world. Sometimes the terms of health education and health promotion are used interchangeably; however, health education has the longest history regarding its extensive mission within society and health care (Penhollow, 2012).

Health Promotion

The Joint Committee on Health Education and Promotion Terminology (2012) defines health promotion as "any planned combination of educational, political, environmental, regulatory, or organizational mechanisms that support actions and conditions of living conducive to the health of individuals, groups and communities." O'Donnell (2009) defines health promotion as both art and science combined to help people ". . . discover the synergies between their core passions and optimal health, enhancing their motivation to strive for optimal health, and supporting them in changing their lifestyle to move toward a state of optimal health." He additionally emphasized the important and dynamic balance among physical, emotional, social, spiritual, and intellectual health. The role of health education in health promotion can be observed in lifestyle changes that are facilitated through selected combinations of learning experiences and strategies. Health promotion efforts also seek to enhance awareness, encourage commitment to action, and build needed skills. According to O'Donnell (2009), health promotion's most important contribution is "through the creation of opportunities that open access to environments that make positive health practices the easiest choice."

Health promotion is a broad field encompassing educational, social, economic, and political efforts to improve the health of a population, emerging as an unifying concept bringing a number of separate fields under one umbrella. Health promotion enables people to take control and responsibility for their health, requires close cooperation of heterogeneous sectors, and combines diverse methods or approaches, while encouraging effective and concrete public participation. Many of the strategies in health promotion come from an ecological perspective that seeks to empower individuals, groups, communities in developing behaviors and lifestyles that enhance health.

Health promotion is made up of three important areas of practice, each of which has a vital role in achieving health for the individual and the community: health education, health protection, and disease prevention. These are commonly referred to as the triad of health promotion. The professionals in these areas of practice work together providing the best opportunities for individuals, groups, and communities to make choices for optimal health.

Health Education

Health education is at the core of total health promotion programming. Health education professionals provide knowledge, skill development, and support that help clients understand their options and voluntarily choose health behaviors for optimal health and high quality of life. While other professions are involved in the work of health promotion, health education is the primary profession devoted to health promotion and whose practitioners are trained in a range of health promotion processes (Simons-Morton, Greens, & Gottlieb, 1995). Health education is a planned process which usually combines educational experiences to facilitate voluntary adaptations or establishment of behavior conducive to health. Health education specialists educate individuals about their own health as well as educate the media, elected officials, and community leaders.

Disease Prevention

Disease prevention is a major emphasis for health promotion. Disease prevention, according to the Joint Committee (2012), "is the process of reducing risks and alleviating disease to promote, preserve, and restore health and minimize suffering and distress." Prevention consists of three levels of prevention. Each has specific implications for the health education specialist or health promoter. Each requires different objectives, methods, and interventions (programs).

Primary prevention emphasizes interventions to avert disease, illness, injury, or deterioration of health before these occur. Primary prevention may include vaccinations and immunizations for children and adults. Vaccinations will cause the production of antibodies which will prevent future cases of a disease so that people will not get sick.

Another example of primary prevention is early pregnancy interventions that teach pregnant women to adopt healthy behaviors that support healthy pregnancies, deliveries, and healthy newborns. There are legislative actions that are considered primary prevention, such as water fluoridation, seat belt laws, laws requiring child restraint seats in vehicles, laws requiring immunizations before attending school, and laws requiring food handlers to be periodically tested for infectious diseases. All of these actions are designed to prevent diseases, disabilities, and injuries. It is at the primary prevention level that health education specialists and health promoters can have their greatest impact on the health of a population. Primary prevention is the most cost-effective form of disease prevention.

Secondary prevention identifies diseases at their earliest stages and applies appropriate measures to limit the consequences and severity of the disease. The efforts in secondary prevention center on early detection and treatment of diseases. The focus is curative and this has been the primary focus for medicine. Secondary prevention directs resources to identify diseases at the earliest stage possible so that the damage from the disease can be limited. Examples of secondary prevention are mammograms, Pap tests, testicular exams, regular blood pressure measurements, measurements for blood cholesterol and blood glucose, and vision examinations. The health education specialist or patient educator in many of these situations plays an important role in getting clients to schedule tests for early detection of diseases and for providing the knowledge and skills for clients to reduce or avoid the destructive disease progress and improve their health.

Tertiary prevention helps people who already have diseases and disabilities. Tertiary prevention prescribes specific interventions to limit the effects of disabilities and diseases and may also prevent the recurrence of disease. The level of tertiary prevention will depend on the medical care that is available to the individual or community. Some of the critical components of tertiary care are rehabilitation services, physical therapy, and occupational therapy that may not be available to individuals because of costs or lack of health insurance, or because such services are not available in some communities. This level of tertiary prevention will depend heavily on surgery, medications, and counseling. Tertiary prevention and the care required at this level is the most expensive, when compared to secondary or primary prevention. It is the least cost-effective in preventing illness and disease.

Health Protection

Health protection includes ". . . the legal or fiscal controls, other regulations and policies, and voluntary codes of practice, aimed at the enhancement of positive health and the prevention of ill health" (Downie et. al., 1996). Health education specialists and promoters must overcome many barriers to health protection. The mission of health protection is to provide legislative, political, and social constructs that reduce the likelihood of people behaving in unsafe ways or to remove environmental hazards that impact health outcomes. Rules that forbid smoking in the workplace, laws that tax tobacco products, and regulations forbidding smoking in schools and other public places are all examples of health protections that have reduced smoking among some populations and reduced the likelihood that these populations will develop certain cancers or cardiovascular diseases. Many efforts to establish and enforce health protection have met with great opposition because it violates one of the tenets of health education and health promotion: individuals have the constitutional right to voluntarily choose to change behaviors that promote health. This opposition to certain efforts for health protection is found among lobbying organizations, political groups, and industries, with just as many groups and organizations supporting these efforts.

The Triad of Health Promotion

Tannahill (1985) noted that these three areas that make up health promotion generate seven domains. As the health professionals in disease prevention, health education, and health protection relate to, intersect, and interact with each other, the following seven domains arise in health promotion.

Figure 2.1 The seven domains produced by triad of health promotion

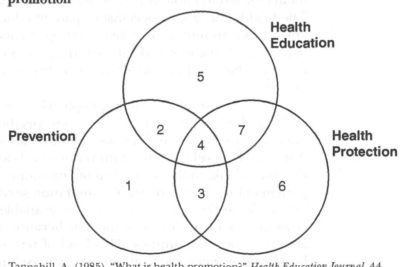

Tannahill, A. (1985). "What is health promotion?" *Health Education Journal*, 44, 167–8.

1. Prevention:
   This domain includes the primary, secondary, and tertiary prevention measures and programs.

2. Lifestyle:
   This domain results from the interaction of disease prevention and health education. It is comprised of educational efforts to influence lifestyle to prevent health problems and to encourage participation in preventive services.

3. Preventive Policies:
   This domain results from the interaction of disease prevention and health protection. This domain represents preventive health protection. Examples of the work in this domain would be water purification, water fluoridation, restaurant inspections, etc. The domain would be considered to be policy commitments to preventive efforts under domain 1.

4. Policy Maker Education:
   The interactions among disease prevention, health education, and health protection gives rise to professionals and services that are involved in preparing and stimulating the social environment, legislators, and policy makers to support preventive health protection actions and measures.

5. Health Education:
   This domain involves all aspects of health education that influences health behaviors for positive health outcomes.

6. Health Protection:
   This domain supports the implementation of policies and the commitment of funds for health protection efforts.

7. Policy Support:
   This domain is an interaction of health education and health protection. It involves a policy commitment to positive health and raising awareness and securing support for positive health protection measures among the public and policy makers.

Primary Themes in Health Promotion

Health promotion seeks improved health and quality of life for the individual, but also for groups and the general population. In observing the many health promotion interventions and strategies, it becomes obvious that there are specific themes in health promotion efforts. Some of these themes are listed below (Butler, 2001).

- Empowerment:
  Empowerment is a multilevel construct that involves people assuming control over their lives in the context of their social and political environment.

- Ecological Perspective:
  The ecological perspective views health as a product of the inter-dependence of the individual and subsystems of the ecosystem such as family, culture, and physical and social environment.

- Community Organization:
  Community organization is a multi-phased process by which community groups are helped to produce change and develop their community for improved health and quality of life.

- Individual Behavior:
  Although we emphasize social and economic factors, we must not forget the crucial role of individual behavior in one's health.

- Official Recognition:
  Many official United States, Canadian, and international pronouncements have recognized the importance of health promotion and have laid a groundwork for its continued growth.

References

Butler, J. T. 2001. *Principles of Health Education and Health Promotion,* 3rd ed. Belmont, CA: Wadsworth/Thomson Learning.

Downie, R. S., C. Tannahill, and A. Tannahill. 1996. *Health Promotion: Models and Values,* 2nd ed. Oxford, England: Oxford University Press.

Doyle, E., and S. Ward. 2005. *The Process of Community Health Education and Promotion.* Long Grove, IL: Waveland Press, Inc.

Gochman, D. S. 1982. "Labels, Systems, and Motives: Some Perspectives on Future Research." *Health Education Quarterly* 9: 167–74.

Gochman, D. S. 1997. "Health Behavior Research: Definitions and Diversity." In D. S. Gochman (Ed.), *Handbook of Health Behavior Research: Vol.1. Personal and Social Determinants.* New York: Plenum Press.

Green, L. W., and M. W. Kreuter. 1999. *Health Promotion Planning: An Educational and Ecological Approach,* 3rd ed. Mountain View, CA: Mayfield.

Joint Committee on Health Education and Promotion Terminology. 2012. "Report of the 2011 Joint Committee on Health Education and Promotion Terminology." *American Journal of Health Education* 43 (2).

McGinnis, J. M., P. Williams-Russo, and J. R. Knickman. 2002. "The case for more active policy attention to health promotion." *Health Affairs* 21 (2): 78–93.

Oberteuffer, D., O. A. Harrelson, and M. B. Pollock. 1972. *School Health Education,* 5th ed. New York: Harper & Row.

O'Donnell Michael P. 2009. "Definition of Health Promotion 2.0: Embracing Passion, Enhancing Motivation, Recognizing Dynamic Balance, and Creating Opportunities." *American Journal of Health Promotion: September/October 2009* 24 (1): iv.

Penhollow, T. M. 2012. *Points to Health: Theory and Practice of Health Education and Health Behavior.* Dubuque, IA: Kendall Hunt Publishing Company.

Simons-Morton, B. G., W. H. Greens, and N. H. Gottlieb. 1995. *Introduction to Health Education and Health Promotion,* 2nd ed. Prospects Heights, IL: Waveland.

Tannahill, A. 1985. What is Health Promotion? *Health Education Journal* 44: 167–8.

Chapter 3

A Historical Context for Health Education and Health Promotion

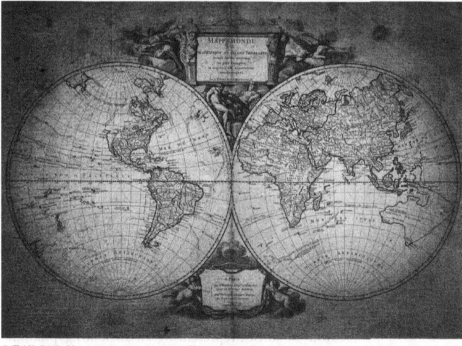

This chapter presents a brief overview of history as it leads to the development of the health education profession. It is not meant to be an exhaustive account but allows the reader to examine some of the events and developments that have led to the field and practice of health education and health promotion. Health education and promotion share the same historical roots as many other health professions that lead in protecting the health of populations. This history started with the beginning of civilization. Historical and archaeological evidence reveals a preoccupation by people with their survival. Acquiring behaviors and developing rules and regulations that protect people's health have been major factors in the development of civilizations throughout the world. Humans have investigated and determined, to the best of their abilities and resources, how to be safe and healthy, avoiding injuries, sickness, and premature death. Historically, health information has been passed from person to person in a variety of ways, starting with word-of-mouth, the oral traditions, traditional customs, and spiritual and religious beliefs and practices.

Early Civilizations

Ancient writings and records reflect varied approaches for medicine and public health. Much of what earlier cultures and societies learned and accomplished resulted from trial and error, scientific exploration and research, and through spiritual and religious beliefs and practices. In fact, in earlier societies, there were strong associations among sciences and religion and spiritual beliefs in supporting health for the individual and the communities. In many early cultures, priests or spiritual leaders served as physicians (Ferngren, 2009).

This history of health care similarly is reflected in many civilizations and cultures throughout the world. There are many documented efforts for the protection of the population's health. Early efforts at public health are identified by existing evidence of bathrooms and drain systems in the Indus Valley dating back at least 4,000 years. The ancient kingdoms of Africa such as Egypt and Mali and those of China were noted for their advanced knowledge in medicine and surgeries in many archaeological finds.

Smith Papyri documents Africa's early contribution to health care. The Smith Papyri is the oldest written documents related to health care dating from 3000 BC, representing an ancient Egyptian medical textbook on surgery (U.S. National Library of Medicine, n.d.). It begins with clinical cases of head injuries and works systematically down the body, describing, in detail, the examination, diagnosis, treatment, and prognosis in each case. It reveals the ancient Egyptians' knowledge of the relation of the pulse to the heart and of the workings of the stomach, bowels, and larger blood vessels. Historically, the first physician of notable reputation was Imhotep, who existed at least 1,000 years before the Greek Hippocrates. Monuments to Imhotep's wisdom, medical expertise and power still stand in Egypt today.

A major document for health laws in the Babylonian Empire is in the Code of Hammurabi, which dates back to about 1772 BC. The sixth

Babylonian king, Hammurabi, enacted the code, which exists on a human-sized stone *stele* with various clay tablets. The Code consists of 282 laws, some of which deal with punishments and also contains directives and rules for health practices and physicians, including the first known fee schedule for health services (Butler, 2001).

Judeo-Christian history contributes many formal directions for health and the quality of life in the tenets of Judaism and Christianity that illustrated the close relationship of spiritual beliefs and practices with health practices and regulations. Throughout the Pentateuch of the Old Testament, especially the Book of Leviticus, the Hebrews are directed by God on how to live holy and healthy lives through spiritual practices, sanitation, care of the sick, childbirth, dietary directives, and burial practices. The early Christian church during the Roman Empire made important innovations with patient care for the sick with the establishment of hospital and nursing care (Guenter, 1999; Ferngren, 2009).

The ancient Greeks placed great emphasis on prevention rather than treatment of disease. They actually compartmentalized the aspects of physical, mental, and spiritual health, but maintained the importance of balancing these aspects of health. Greeks believed in the perfect balance of mind, body, and spirit, actualized through the study and practice of philosophy, athletics, and theology. Greek mythology played a significant role in the history of health in Greek culture. In the classic, *The Iliad*, a Thesalian chief named Asclepius received instruction in use of drugs and was later endowed as the god of medicine. He had two daughters Hygeia and Panacea. Hygeia was given the ability to prevent disease. Panacea was given the ability to treat disease. The words *hygiene* and *panacea* traced back to these mythical daughters of Asclepius. Throughout Greece, temples were erected to worship the mythical god Asclepius. The caduceus, the symbol of the staff and serpent of the physician, was an important symbol of these temples. Hippocrates was a famous and authentic Greek physician who practiced medicine in the Asclepian tradition. Hippocrates was known for his approach to medicine that included observing and recording associations between certain diseases and factors such as geography, climate, diet, and living conditions. He was able to distinguish endemic diseases and epidemic diseases. The Hippocratic Oath still serves as the basis for medical ethics in the western world today. Hippocrates is also considered to be the first epidemiologist and the father of modern medicine.

The Roman Empire conquered the Greeks and many other kingdoms, but did not destroy their cultures; they expanded them. The Romans brought the ancient world great engineers, builders, and administrators. The Romans built an extensive and efficient aqueduct system. They developed an extensive system of underground sewers and public and private baths. These great innovations made sanitary and healthful environments possible. Roman civilization developed a system of private medical practice. They expanded the study of anatomy and surgery that began with the Greeks (Rosen, 1958).

The Pre-Modern Era

With the fall of the Roman Empire, many of the advances in western medicine and public health were lost. Without the power of Rome and the invasions of barbarian hordes, great fear existed among Rome's former subjects. This was the period of the Middle Ages which are also referred to as the Dark Ages. Fear drove many people into walled cities for protection. Rosen (1958) describes how people lived with their animals within these cities and how, as the populations grew in these confined areas, sanitation and health broke down. The norms for cleanliness disappeared, replaced by often filthy conditions by the common people and aristocracies. The Roman advances in community health were lost during this period. Superstition and misinterpretation of Christian beliefs led to the destruction of many of the written science and medical advances from the Greeks and Romans. Some few documents were saved by the Christian Church.

It is not surprising that the Middle Ages gave rise to many deadly epidemics. One of the most deadly of all diseases was the Black Death or bubonic plague. It is estimated that the bubonic plague may have claimed more than 30 million lives. Europe may have lost a quarter to one-third of its populations. The cause of the disease was unknown at that time, so great fear and superstition existed around the disease. Often, the first to respond to the people suffering from this disease were the religious leaders and the doctors. This meant that the mortality rate among these practitioners was very high and often left communities with no spiritual or medical leadership (Cottrell, 2012).

Great numbers of lives were lost as those of the Middle Ages grappled with epidemics of the bubonic plague, leprosy, smallpox, diphtheria, measles, influenza, tuberculosis, anthrax, and finally, syphilis (McKenzie et. al., 2008). While there was no agreement about the causes of these diseases, it eventually became clear that contagion might be involved. Education about how to handle the diseases and avoid contracting the diseases became important. While there were no professional health educators at this time, there were professionals that took on this task of educating the public about disease prevention: priests, pastors, medical doctors, and community leaders. They attempted to teach anyone who would listen about how to protect their health, even though the information was limited.

The Middle Ages lasted until about 1500 AD, with the advent of the Renaissance (1500–1700 AD). The disease conditions of the Middles Ages continued, but science began to emerge as a legitimate means of inquiry. Eventually there were many advancements to begin some improvement in the health and quality of life in populations of this time period. It was again deemed appropriate to study the human body. The search for knowledge was renewed. This led to great exploration for new lands and new trade routes. However, in Europe, some problems still persisted. Problems such as the inappropriate disposal of human waste and lack of bathing were prevalent among the poor, the growing middle class, and the aristocracies of the time. While perfume is an ancient tradition, during the

Renaissance, "cloaking scents" were used to cover the bad odors left in clothing (Hansen, 1980).

As many of the superstitions of the Middle Ages were being replaced by observations of cause and effect, there were numerous advances in health care during this period. Through his orderly study of the human body, John Hunter became known as the father of modern surgery. The invention of the microscope by Antoine van Leeuwenhoek enabled mankind to see life forms too small to be seen by the naked eye. However, this new science was not associated with discovery of disease. John Graunt expanded the fields of biostatistics and epidemiology with his studies and publications on mortality (Goerke and Stebbins, 1968, p.61). Cipolla (1976) found that many Italian cities had established boards of health to fight the communicable diseases, but by the middle of the sixteenth century their control and jurisdiction expanded to include the food trade, wine, water, the sewage systems, the hospital practices, burials, cemeteries, as well as the professional practices of physicians, surgeons, and pharmacies. These boards of health even had jurisdiction over beggars and prostitutes.

The New World

Explorers had come to North America from all over the world for many centuries. When Europeans arrived in North America, they found generally healthy populations of American Indians. Among American Indian nations, health information and healing practices were passed from generation to generation by traditional practices and word-of-mouth. They were not prepared for the life threatening challenges that would come from Europe. Arrival of Europeans to North America brought new diseases and epidemics to the American Indians as well as to the colonists who had settled in the New World for a new life. The new life was fraught with many hardships, dangers, and challenges. Diseases and epidemics would destroy whole settlements of colonists and whole communities of American Indians. Perhaps smallpox was one of the deadliest diseases impacting these people. There was little experience or expertise to deal with the overwhelming challenges to life. Community health action in the colonies was usually ineffective, and taken only in crises. The practice of medicine was primitive.

In the Massachusetts colony, there was legislation passed in 1701 to provide isolation and quarantine practices for those who suffered from smallpox. As various cultures and nations fought the spread of disease and major epidemics, it became apparent to some leaders that such disease and health challenges with the accompanying unsanitary conditions in many areas could be alleviated with organized community efforts and improving the educational levels of the people. Many of the colonies in the New World followed the community health actions in Europe by establishing several local boards of health in the late 1790s due to yellow fever epidemics. In 1746, the Massachusetts Bay colonies passed laws for the prevention of pollution in the Boston Harbor.

Harvard College became the first institution of higher education in the colonies, founded in 1636, before compulsory schooling for children was installed. Harvard offered the first required hygiene course in American higher education. In early America, only boys went to school. In 1642, Massachusetts became the first colony to establish a law requiring all children to read and write. Benjamin Franklin advocated health and physical exercise and in 1751 he realized the founding of the first Academy in Philadelphia, the first secondary education in America that also supported these principles. In 1821 the American high school was established.

A Case History of Smallpox in the Ancient and New World

Smallpox is a vicious disease that ravaged all civilizations from antiquities until the 20th century. The smallpox scars on the mummified features of Pharaoh Ramses V testify to the long relationship with this disease, a disease unique to humans and one that has killed millions (Behbehani, 1983). Descriptions of smallpox appear in the earliest Egyptian, Indian, and Chinese writings. Smallpox spread through contact with living sufferers or the bodies of the dead; it was especially cruel on previously unexposed populations—at least one-third of all Aztecs died after Spanish colonizers brought smallpox to the New World in 1518.

Survivors of smallpox carried its legacies for life. Many people were left blind and virtually all survivors were disfigured by scars from the disease. By the 1500s, the disease had reached most of the world and the smallpox scarred faces were familiar sights. The wealthier survivors in Elizabethan society used shaped beauty patches to camouflage the damage or coated their faces with white lead powder. The ghostly pale face of Queen Elizabeth I was as much a sign of her brush with smallpox as it was a fashion statement. Eventually, many survivors of the dreaded disease realized that they had gained an advantage over those who had not experienced smallpox. Their bouts with smallpox yielded lifelong immunity from any further infection from smallpox.

All over the world people were discovering that immunity was not inherited, because an outbreak in one generation in a city did not protect future generations in that city from smallpox. However, in many countries, investigations of the smallpox led to the idea that immunity could be induced through inoculation. The idea of preventing smallpox epidemics by inducing immunity was first exploited in China, where a form of inoculation existed as early as the tenth century. Immunity was gained by provoking a mild form of the disease in healthy people, for example by blowing powdered smallpox scabs up their noses. Other world cultures used varying forms of inoculation to protect its citizens. The form of inoculation for smallpox in Africa became an important weapon against the disease in the New World. By the early 1700s, smallpox inoculation, known as *variolation*, had spread from parts of Africa, India, and the Ottoman Empire. Lady Mary Wortley Montagu, a well-known writer and wife of a wealthy English aristocrat, moved to the Ottoman Empire when her husband was assigned to be ambassador to the Ottoman Empire. While there, Lady Mary Wortley Montagu encountered this smallpox variolation process in 1717. She witnessed local peasant women performing inoculations or variolations at seasonal 'smallpox parties'. Upon returning to Britain, she had her own children inoculated during an outbreak in 1721.

Even with Lady Montagu's campaigning on behalf of inoculation, the British were reluctant to adopt this practice to thwart the devastation of smallpox. In 1721, at the urging of Montagu and the Princess of Wales, several prisoners and abandoned children were inoculated by having smallpox inserted under the skin. Several months later, the children and prisoners who were deliberately exposed to smallpox did not develop the smallpox disease. When none contracted the disease, the procedure was deemed safe and members of the royal family were inoculated. The procedure then became fashionable in Europe.

While the slave trade in the New World was horrific, evil, and inhumane, it was the African slaves who introduced variolation into America. In Massachusetts, Cotton Mather learned about the practice from his slave, Onesimus, who had received the treatment as a child in Africa. Onesimus was immune from smallpox and so were many other slaves as Mather discovered as he investigated this fully (Herbert, 1975). Mather publicized the technique and the procedure was first tried during the smallpox epidemic in Boston in 1721. Inspired by Onesimus's knowledge, Mather campaigned for inoculation in the face of the growing epidemic, a call that met with some success and much hostility. However, the actions of Lady Montagu, the knowledge of Onesimus, and the persistence of Cotton Mather ultimately hastened this knowledge transfer to the Western world. Edward Jenner, an English country doctor, later adapted the practice, and developed a safer, more effective technique he called vaccination. He noted that local people who caught cowpox gained immunity from the far more dangerous smallpox. Jenner's relentless promotion and devoted research of vaccination changed the way medicine was practiced. Late in the 19th century, it was realized that vaccination did not confer lifelong immunity and that subsequent revaccination was necessary.

The mortality from smallpox had declined, but there were still epidemics, showing that the disease was still not under control. In the 1950s a number of control measures were implemented, and smallpox was eradicated in many areas in Europe and North America. In 1967, a global campaign began under the direction of the World Health Organization and finally succeeded in the eradication of smallpox in 1977. On May 8, 1980, the World Health Assembly announced that the world was free of smallpox and recommended that all countries cease vaccination (Riedel, 2005).

Pre-Industrial Era (1800–1850)

The United States was swept by a series of epidemics and physicians were poorly trained. Medical problems were addressed by poorly prepared physicians with unsanitary conditions. There were many political and social problems that led to changes in education. States gradually made education mandatory and health education principles and policies were starting to form. William Alcott, the father of school health education in the United States, wrote an important book on the healthful construction of schoolhouses, and he was the first to write a health book for children. Horace Mann was the first secretary of the first board of education in the United States. Horace Mann was also one of the most influential educators of his day. He made powerful recommendations for physiology and hygiene in the curriculum of the elementary school, resulting in the mandatory addition of these subjects to the curriculum of all public schools in 1850 in Massachusetts.

As communities became more industrialized in England, health and living conditions plummeted especially with the working poor. Edwin Chadwick published the *Report on the Inquiry into the Sanitary Condition of the Labouring Population in Great Britain* in 1842. The report described the wretched conditions of Great Britain's working class in both their homes and in the workplaces. With much opposition, Chadwick proposed that political unrest and poverty were not the most critical contributors to the poor health, but the filth and the immorality of the poor were the primary and direct causes of poor personal and community health, family discord, and alcohol abuse among this population (Rosen, 1993; Hamlin 1995). Chadwick's work led to the 1848 Public Health Act and the establishment of the General Board of Health in England. This organization authorized local boards of health to oversee the water supply, sewage, and to conduct surveys and investigations of sanitary conditions in given districts.

Chadwick's work had far reaching implications for public health practice that impacted not only England, but also impacted public health foundations in the United States. In the United States, Lemuel Shattuck published the *Report of the Sanitary Commission of Massachusetts* in 1850. This report publicized and supported community health promotion and it served as a guide in the health field for a century. The report made fifty recommendations that were established in public health practice. Shattuck's report helped society address health problems in a more disciplined way and endorsed an ambitious program of health education in schools.

The Modern Era: 1850–Present

Report on the Inquiry into Sanitary Condition of the Labouring Population of Great Britain (Edwin Chadwick, 1842) and *Report of the Sanitary Commission of Massachusetts* (Lemuel Shattuck, 1850) ushered in the modern era of health.

Society began to attack health problems in a disciplined way, even though there were some false assumptions. The modern era of health has been divided into five phases that reflect the foci and beliefs about community health during these periods, but not always with accurate science and evidence. Each of these phases were marked by various major advances in the health of populations, medical and public health innovations, educational programming, and the importance of health education and health promotion in personal and public health improvements. These phases include the following:

- Miasma Phase (1850–1880)
- Bacteriology Phase (1880–1910)
- Health Resources Phase (1910–1960)
- Social Engineering Phase (1960–1975)
- Health Promotion Phase (1970s–Present)

The Miasma Phase (1850–1880)

Miasma refers to toxic vapors or fumes. During the miasma phase, people thought that disease was caused by toxic vapors. The effect of quarantine and isolation led to the mistaken assumption that confining the unhealthy air that carried disease was beneficial in preventing the disease. It was believed that the use of herbs and incense to perfume the air and the body would "fill the nose and crowd out the miasma.

Local and state powers were directed to the fight against infectious diseases. The American Public Health Association was founded in 1872. Florence Nightingale actively defined laws for nursing and developed the concept of nursing as a profession. The Women's Christian Temperance Movement, very strong scientific temperance movement, preached the evils of alcohol and other drugs, forced passage of many laws requiring instruction on the effects of drugs and hygiene education in 38 states between 1880 and 1890. The American Medical Association (AMA) was founded on May 7, 1847.

Bacteriology Phase (1880–1910)

The bacteriology phase was ushered in by the work of such scientists as Louis Pasteur and Robert Koch, presenting evidence that microorganisms cause infectious diseases. This information was not readily accepted, so the nineteenth century ended with major epidemics and the primary tools used in the attacks on these diseases were still isolation and quarantine.

The physical education movement began in this period, pioneered by Catherine Esther Beecher and Thomas Denison Wood. Their work laid some of the foundation for health education. During this era of medical inspection, physicians and health workers examined school children and teachers to identify those whose health problems made them dangerous to others in efforts to reduce the incidences of communicable diseases. The Modern Health Crusade of the National Tuberculosis Association was a multiphasic program to encourage healthy behaviors in school children. School children were encouraged to practice several health chores daily and various levels of achievement were rewarded and recognized. The campaign for "open-air classrooms" provided open-air schools and classrooms, usually in hospital settings, that provided fresh air and an opportunity to integrate health education into the overall education plan for children with tuberculosis.

Health Resources Phase (1910–1960)

With the growing recognition of the importance of health education in preventing and addressing diseases came much social reform that improved health in United States. John Upton's book *The Jungle* revealed the deplorable working conditions of immigrants working in the meat packing industry and the contamination of food. This led to the passage of the Pure Food and Drug Act of 1906 and the passage of workman's compensation laws. During the health resources phase, large financial investments were made in hospitals, health staffing, and biomedical research.

Until 1910, health education, hygiene education, and physical education were considered synonymous (Anderson, 1972). Then the American Physical Education Association recognized the difference between hygiene education and health education, professionally separating the two. Most degree programs offered training in physical education and hygiene. However, the Health Department of the Georgia Normal and Industrial College became the first institution to offer a curriculum and an undergraduate degree in health education in 1921. This was followed by the Teachers College of Columbia University and the Harvard University-Massachusetts Institute of Technology combined program awarding degrees in health education. The *Cardinal Principles of Secondary Education*, published by the National Education Association (NEA) in 1918, marked a turning point in United States secondary education and legitimized school health education. In 1918, the Child Health Organization was founded in response to concerns about childhood malnutrition and is often considered the beginning of the health education movement. Health education curriculum changed during the 1920s due, in part, to the Report of the Joint Committee on Health Problems in Education published by the NEA and the AMA, *A Survey of 86 Cities*, showing that health education across the country was not consistent. Health education became the focus of several commercial companies and industries that produced high quality curricula and audiovisual materials to be utilized in health education efforts. The American School Health Association was founded in 1927. A number of research studies conducted during this period provided a science base for health education.

The Great Depression struck during this phase and impacted every aspect of the American society, even in education and health care. The Depression resulted in program cuts and educational reconstruction, but it was followed by a period of tremendous medical advances and federal investments in the health care system. A series of important conferences, including a series of White House Conferences on Child Health and Protection focused attention on the health of children and the roles of the schools and communities in protecting it.

Social Engineering Phase (1960–1975)

During this phase, there was recognition that not everyone in American society benefited from the educational, technological, and health advances realized at this time. The social engineering phase began in the 1960s, emphasizing and assuring equal access to educational and health services to all citizens regardless of race, ethnicity, and socioeconomic status. Programs such as "New Frontier" and "War on Poverty," were administered to address social wrongs. However, the most significant services to be established by legislation were Medicare and Medicaid in 1965. These programs were amendments to the Social Security Act of 1935 and addressed the needs of two groups who were not likely to have health insurance and health coverage: the elderly and the poor. These programs by law did not allow for discrimination in the provision of health care and quality of services. The School Health Education Study, completed in the mid-1960s, was the first attempt to define what children and youth in the United States knew about health. The results would be used to scientifically develop a health education curriculum following basic principles used for all other educational curricula. During the 1970s, health education moved away from the emphasis on acquisition of facts to more emphasis on the affective domain and later to health behavior choices. The federal government's priority became the cost containment of health care. The Coalition of National Health Education Organizations was established in 1972.

Health Promotion Phase (1970s–Present)

As cost containment for growing health care costs became the priority of the federal government, the focus on changing health behavior also grew as a priority in health education. There was growing understanding that helping individuals establish or make more responsible health behavior choices would lead to greater prevention of costly health problems. The health promotion phase has focused on innovative programming to change behaviors that pose health risks and to encourage behaviors that are beneficial to health. The Society for Public Health Education (SOPHE) published the first genuine code of ethics for health educators in 1976 AAHE adopted the AAHE Code of Ethics in 1993. There was a call for all health education organizations to develop a profession-wide code of ethics. After much commitment and work, in November 1999, delegates of the Ethics Task Force of the Coalition of National Health Education Organizations (CNHEO) approved the most recent Code of Ethics for the Health Education Profession.

The Lalonde Report, *A New Perspective on the Health of Canadians* introduced the "health field" concept that identified four elements to which death and disease could be attributed: human biology (heredity), environment, lifestyle (behavior), and inadequacies in health care provision. The Lalonde report directly influenced the health promotion movement in the United States. The US government published several documents recognizing the importance of lifestyle in promoting health and well-being (US Public Health Service, 1979). The US government through the leadership of the US Surgeon General embarked upon the challenge to set a national agenda that communicated a common vision for improving health and achieving health equity. The series of publications include *Healthy People: The Surgeon General's Report on Health Promotion and Disease Prevention* (1979), *Promoting Health/Preventing Disease: Objectives for the Nation* (1980), *Healthy People 2000* (1990), *Healthy People 2010* (2000), and the more recent *Healthy People 2020* (2010). These all have called attention to the roles of individuals, their communities, and their governments in supporting health. Each publication provided measurable health objectives for the nation to meet overarching national goals within a given ten-year timeframe.

Table 3.1 Healthy People 2020; Vision, Mission, and Goals

Vision: A society in which all people live long, healthy lives.
Mission: Healthy People 2020 strives to: • identify nationwide health improvement priorities   • increase public awareness and understanding of the determinants of health, disease, disability, and the opportunities for progress   • provide measurable objectives and goals that are applicable at the national, state, and local levels   • engage multiple sectors to take actions to strengthen policies and improve practices that are driven by the best available evidence and knowledge.   • identify critical research, evaluation, and data collection needs.
Overarching Goals: • Attain high-quality, longer lives free of preventable disease, disability, injury, and premature death;   • Achieve health equity, eliminate disparities, and improve the health of all groups;   • Create social and physical environments that promote good health for all;   • Promote quality of life, healthy development, and healthy behaviors across all life stages.

Source: Centers for Disease Control and Prevention, Healthy People 2020.

There have been and continue to be several international conferences that support and nurture the health promotion movement in a global context as well. The HIV+/AIDS epidemics beginning in the 1970's and continuing currently, major natural disasters and international terrorism continue to emphasize the need to work through health education and health promotion to assess health needs, encourage positive behavior changes, plan effective programs for disease prevention, health protection, and to evaluate these efforts to improve methods, strategies and outcomes.

The decades of the 1990s and 2000s have focused on the ecological perspective, taking into account the social, political, and economic forces impacting and affecting health. Butler (2001) suggests that this era, 1990s through the present, may be known in the future as the beginning of the phase of social ecology.

In March 23, 2010, amid much controversy, the Affordable Care Act became national law. The intention of the law is to expand health care coverage to 31 million uninsured Americans. The law will also focus on prevention and prevention services through community and wellness programs, worksite wellness programs and strong support for school-based health centers. Time will tell if these goals will be realized for the American people.

Professional Credentialing

The potential for making our society healthier with the practices of responsible health behaviors has seldom been greater for health education specialists and those working in health promotion. With the evolution of health education as a profession, there has been debate over the qualifications necessary for successful health education and health promotion practice. The process of identifying the competencies of professional health educators began in 1948 with the National Conference on Undergraduate Professional Preparation in Health Education, Physical Education and Recreation. In 1962, the American Association for Health, Physical Education and Recreation identified seven areas upon which principles and standards for health education were centered and for which professional competencies were identified.

As a result of the First Bethesda Conference in 1978, the National Task Force on the Preparation and Practice of Health Education was given the responsibility of developing a credentialing system for health education. This resulted in the Role Delineation Project which identified the responsibilities, tasks, and competencies of practicing health educators. Next, the Role Delineation Project established the concept of a generic health educator, regardless of title, audience or setting, and the required competencies and skills of such a professional. The competencies and skills for entry-level health educators were defined in *A Guide for the Development of Competency-Based Curricula for Entry-Level Health Educators* in 1981. This became a resource document that was revised and retitled *A Competency*

Based Curriculum Framework for the Professional Preparation of Entry-Level Health Educators.

In 1988, the National Commission on Health Education Credentialing, Inc. (NCHEC) was established to promote and sustain a body of credentialed health education professionals. NCHEC monitors and awards the Certified Health Education Specialist credential, certifying health education specialists, promoting professional development and enhancing professional preparation and practice (National Commission for Health Education Credentialing, 2012).

Summary

This brief historical account of health, public health, and health promotion takes the reader through many different periods of time and stages of health conditions in the world and in the United States. We have seen the plight of humans as they dealt with disease and epidemics in the past when primarily all health efforts were focused on preventing or avoiding disease and early death to the current times when there is greater emphasis on promoting health and improving the quality of life for all citizens. It has been interesting to follow the transitions from Lemuel Shattuck's era in Boston, when tuberculosis was raging and the average age of death decreased from 27.85 years in 1820–1825 to 21.43 years in 1840–1845. In New York, over the same time periods the average age of death decreased from 26.15 years to 19.69 (Butler, 2001). By the 1900s, life expectancy in the United States was 49.24 years, and by the 1990s, life expectancy had risen to 76.1. In 2007, US life expectancy reached 77.9 years (CDC/NCHS, n.d.). Many of the factors that contributed to this improved health status and increasing life span in the United States are due to many health and medical advances, an explosion of new knowledge and practices that protect and promote health, the conquering of many life-threatening communicable diseases, improved and safer food sources, and populations making better health choices. However, the successes that have improved the health of the American people may mask health challenges that are still causing disabilities and premature death for high risk populations. Still, poor socioeconomic conditions, discrimination, and health inequities in this country are impacting the health of significant numbers of people in the United States. Many of the current challenges are related to health and lifestyle choices and behaviors. More than 40 percent of the primary causes of death are directly impacted by health behaviors and lifestyle choices. The primary causes of death are lifestyle diseases. The work before those in health education and health promotion is great in this country and in the world.

References

Anderson, C. I. 1972. *School Health Policies.* St. Louis: C.V. Mosby.

Behbehani, Abbas M. 1983. "The Smallpox Story: Life and Death of an Old Disease." *Microbiological Reviews* 47 (4): 455–509.

Butler, J. T. 2001. *Principles of Health Education and Health Promotion.* Belmont, CA: Wadsworth/Thomson Learning.

Centers for Disease Control and Prevention, Healthy People. 2020. Retrieved at: http://www.cdc.gov/nchs/ppt/nchs2012/SS-25_WRIGHT.pdf.

Chadwick, E. 1842/1965. *Report on the Inquiry into Sanitary Condition of the Labouring Population of Great Britain.* Edinburgh, Scotland: Edinburgh University Press.

Cottrell, R. R., J. T. Girvan, and J. F. McKenzie. 2012. *Principles and Foundations of Health Promotion and Education.* Boston: Benjamin Cummings.

Ferngren, G. B. 2009. *Medicine and health care in Early Christianity.* Baltimore: The Johns Hopkins University Press.

Guenter, B. R. 1999. *Mending Bodies, Saving Souls: A History of Hospitals.* Oxford, England: Oxford University Press.

Herbert, E. 1975. "Smallpox Inoculation in Africa." *The Journal of African History* 16 (4): 539–59.

McClellan, J. E., and H. Dorn. 2006. *Science and Technology in World History: An Introduction.* Baltimore, MD: Johns Hopkins University.

Riedel, S. 2005. "Edward Jenner and the History of Smallpox and Vaccination." *Baylor University Medical Center Proceedings 2005* 18 (1): 21–25.

Rosen, G. 1958. *A History of Public Health.* New York: MD Publications

Rosen, G. 1993. *A History of Public Health.* Baltimore, MD: Johns Hopkins University Press.

Shattuck, L. 1948. *Report of the Sanitary Commission of Massachusetts, 1850.* New York: Cambridge University Press. (Original published in 1850)

US Public Health Service. 1979. *Healthy People: The Surgeon General's Report on Health Promotion and Disease Prevention.* Washington, DC: US Government Printing Office.

US National Library of Medicine. *Turning the Page Online. The Edwin Smith Surgical Papyrus.* Retrieved May 23, 2014, from http://www.nlm.nih/.../tu

US National Library of Medicine. *Smallpox: A Great and Terrible Scourge.* Retrieved from http://www.nlm.nih.gov/exhibition/smallpox/sp_variolation.html.

Chapter 4

The Health Education and Health Promotion Professional

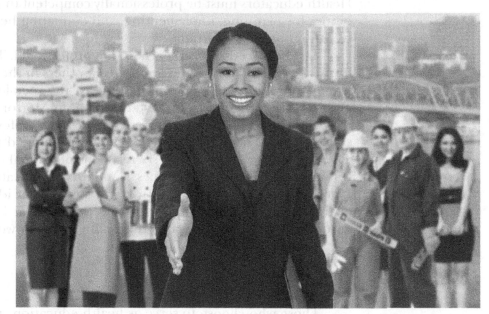

© Kurhan, 2013. Used under license from Shutterstock, Inc.

According to the Joint Committee on Health Education and Health Promotion Terminology (2012), the health educator is a "professionally prepared individual who serves in a variety of roles and is specifically trained to use appropriate educational strategies and methods to facilitate the development of policies, procedures, interventions, and systems conducive to the health of individuals, groups, and communities." A similar but more detailed definition of the health educator is recorded by the U.S. Bureau of Labor Statistics (2012): health educators "promote, maintain, and improve individual and community health by assisting individuals and communities to adopt healthy behaviors. . ." The Bureau of Labor Statistics then describes some of the duties of the health educator as collecting and analyzing data to assess individual and community needs and then using the data to plan, implement, monitor and evaluate programs that encourage healthy lifestyle choices, policies and environments. The health educator is a resource to individuals, communities and other organizations for encouraging associations that support health. The health educator may also manage the fiscal aspects of programs and services. Health educators must be professionally competent in taking on responsibilities for planning, implementing, and evaluating health education and health promotion programs.

The health education specialist is a professional. To be a professional means being held to specific standards by others in the field or profession. Livengood (1996) defined a profession as "the sociological construct for an occupation that has special status." Simons-Morton et. al. (1995) state that there are three essential characteristics of a profession: a service mission, a unique body of knowledge, and a prolonged period of training. These three are supported by six related professional characteristics: continuing education, code of ethics, standards of education, shaping of legislation, freedom from lay control, and strength of identity. All of these characteristics do indeed apply to the professional health educator, regardless of the setting in which the health educator works.

The Mission

Those who choose to serve as health education specialists fulfill the important mission of promoting the health of individuals and communities. Health education specialists have the training and commitment to work with individuals to establish responsible health promoting behaviors. They also work in a larger context to improve the various social conditions that people must deal with to be healthy. Often their efforts are administered in public health facilities, schools, community organizations, faith-based organizations, worksites, etc. While other workers and volunteers may claim to carry out such responsibilities, health education specialists have long term commitment to the profession and to those that they serve, based on essential academic preparation and ongoing experiences to enrich the knowledge and skills needed to effectively help others promote health.

The Body of Knowledge

As indicated in Chapter 2, health education and health promotion have their foundation in a variety of disciplines that support the philosophical base of health education and provide the research base and theoretical framework for establishing and changing health behaviors among a variety of people. The body of knowledge for health education "represents synthesis of facts, principles, and concepts drawn from biological, behavioral, sociological, and health sciences, but interpreted in terms of human needs, human values and human potential" (Cleary et. al., 1996).

The Training Period

While there is agreement in the health education profession on the responsibilities and competencies of the health educator, there is not unanimous agreement on the length of the required training. Required training may vary due to the practice settings of the health education specialists. Those who practice in a school setting are required to have at least a bachelor's degree and state certification and practice as a school teacher. Those health education specialists who practice in a public health department may be required to earn a graduate degree.

According to Butler (2001), more than 300 colleges and universities award undergraduate degrees in health education or health promotion. Many of the programs are housed in schools of public health or colleges of education.

The Council on Education for Public Health (CEPH) is an independent agency recognized by the U.S. Department of Education. Its function is to accredit schools or colleges of public health and public health programs offered in settings other than schools of public health. The schools and programs accredited by CEPH prepare students for entry into careers in public health. The primary professional degree offered by these programs or schools is the Master of Public Health (MPH), but other master's and doctoral degrees are offered as well. As of 2012, CEPH accredits 142 schools and programs (50 schools and 92 programs). CEPH is currently, studying the need for accreditation of baccalaureate programs and what its role should be in this process.

Unfortunately, some who work in the capacity of a health educator are not trained to be a health education specialist. Sometimes the position of health educator is assigned to a person who has no previous training or experience in health education. These individuals must be highly motivated to learn on the job of the health education specialist; but some choose not to. This can be disastrous for the agency and the populations that they serve. Some of these misplaced individuals come from other areas of training and assume that their skills can be made to "fit" the profession. This is erroneous thinking. The health education specialist has a very special and specific knowledge base and skill set tailored to the work of changing health behaviors.

Continuing Education

Members of any profession are expected to keep pace with the changes in knowledge and skills in their areas of expertise. This is especially necessary for health education specialists. While participation in continuing education is not a requirement for health education/health promotion practice in many states, the Certified Health Education Specialists are required to participate in continuing education in order to maintain their certification. Obtaining continuing education experiences and credits can be accomplished through multiple opportunities. These opportunities include participation in professional organizations; attendance at local, state, and national conventions and conferences; successfully completing applicable course work in college/university settings; and the reading of current research and practice articles in peer-reviewed journals and other appropriate literature that informs the professional about the areas of expertise.

Code of Ethics

A code of ethics ensures that practitioners in a given profession will adhere to minimum standards, provide clientele with the standards for what they can expect from the professional and helps the professional to know what is considered acceptable in the profession (Thomasma, 1979). Personal values and morality may guide individuals in one's personal daily life, but these may not be sufficient in professional behaviors and decision making. Professional ethics focus on what is right or wrong in the workplace and are public matters (Cottrell et. al., 2012). Ethics has important meanings for the health education specialists due to their relationships with their clients or students, employees, and the profession. As professionals who teach, train, and counsel, health education specialists are expected to practice in ethical manners. How else can these professionals establish trust relationships with those who they serve? As health education specialist are involved in facilitating voluntary health behavior changes among the individuals and/or target populations that they serve, health educators will become more involved in ethical decisions than other educators.

There are specific ethical issues that will challenge the health education specialist in decision making for planning, practice, research and evaluation. There are several theories on ethics and of course not all are in agreement on what are ethical behaviors. While some philosophers see differences in morality and ethics, the author of this text agrees with Cottrell et. al., (2012, p.147) to ". . . use ethical and moral to mean the same thing." Thiroux, (1995, p. 3) reminds us that "The important thing to remember here is that moral, ethical, immoral, and unethical, essentially mean, good, right, bad, wrong, often depending on whether one is referring to people themselves or to their actions." What indeed are the health education specialists' principles, values and standards that help to answer ethical questions or to solve ethical dilemmas in life and in the professional practice? Thiroux (1995), in *Ethics: Theory and Practice*, suggests five basic principles for common moral ground and ethical practice that can apply to any theoretical framework. These include:

1. Value of life
2. Goodness (Rightness)
   a. Nonmaleficence
   b. Beneficence
3. Justice (Fairness)
4. Honesty (Truthfulness)
5. Individual freedom

Value of life: Human beings must revere life and accept death. No life should be ended without strong justification.

Goodness (rightness): Good and right are at the core of every ethical code. "Good" occurs not only in the abstract but can be seen concretely in relations to other human beings. The principle of goodness included the parallel principles of nonmaleficence and beneficence. Nonmaleficence means no infliction of harm or evil to others. This is an obligation to do no harm: not inflicting harm, removing harm, and preventing harm for others. Beneficence means that there is a responsibility simply to do good. Balog et. al., (1985) said that beneficence "is generally thought to be more altruistic and more far reaching than nonmaleficence because it requires that we take positive steps to help others" (pp. 91–92).

Justice (fairness): Justice relates to treating people fairly and justly in both benefits and burdens. Justice is both procedural and distributive. Procedural justice is whether or not procedures are in place that are fair and whether or not they are being followed for all. Distributive justice relates to the allocation of resources, assuring that everyone has an equal opportunity to obtain the resource or good, and that a person has been given what he or she is due or owed. Tschudin (2003, p. 57) posed the ethical question, "should only those who are able to pay for them receive health education/promotion services, or should only the poor shoulder all of the burden?" (For the health education specialist, this issue is resolved in the Code of Ethics for the Health Education Profession. Article 1, Section 9 states, "Health educators provide services equitably to all people."

Honesty (truthfulness): At the core of any relationship and meaningful communication is telling the truth and being honest. The goal is always to be truthful. However, sometimes a health education specialist may be challenged when there are conflicts of interest. If a minor child asks the health provider for details about his or her health problem and the parents of the minor have instructed the health provider not to engage in such discussions with the minor, the health professional is faced with a conflict of interests. The health professional must address the issue with honesty, honoring the parents' directive.

Individual freedom (equality or autonomy principles): Thiroux (1995) stated "this principle means that people, being individuals with individual differences, must have the freedom to choose their own ways and means of being moral within the framework of the first four principles." (p.187) We must respect others for who they are within the context of the first four principles that Thiroux presented. Health educators are always reminded to respect the rights of others to make their own choices and not to be coerced.

Thiroux's principles are indeed reflected in the *Code of Ethics for the Health Education Profession* found in Appendix A. The Code of Ethics provides the framework grounded in ethical principles and shared values that are foundational for every health education specialist who aspires to the highest standards of conduct in the profession. The Code of Ethics applies to the health education specialists' responsibilities to the public, the profession, in the delivery of health education, in research and evaluation, and in professional preparation. The Code of ethics provides the standards for ethical conduct in the ethical decision making and problem solving processes in health education and health promotion.

Standards of Education

The health education and health promotion areas of emphases on attitudes, lifestyle and behavior change make this profession very different than other disciplines. It is indeed challenging to encourage people to be motivated about behavior change and to address creatively the cultural and social factors affecting health beliefs and behaviors. Add to these challenges the constant scientific and health information changes, it becomes mandatory that health educators remain current in health information and all that transpires in their service populations and communities. Regardless of the setting and the audience there are some competencies and proficiencies that must be present at every level of professional preparation for all health education specialists. There are published responsibilities and competencies that are required for those health education specialists that work in community and public health and for those who are health education specialists in formal educational settings. Anyone preparing for careers in the health education profession must be prepared to fulfill the responsibilities listed in these documents and to demonstrate the competencies supporting the responsibilities. The following two documents will be helpful to the health education student who wants to monitor progress toward fulfilling the competencies and sub-competencies that will prepare him or her to eventually carry out the related responsibilities as a health education specialist or as a school health education teacher.

- *Areas of Responsibilities, Competencies, and Sub-competencies for the Health Education Specialists 2010. (NCHEC) See Appendix B*

- *2008 NCATE Health Education Teacher Preparation Standards. (AAHE) See Appendix C*

Shaping of Legislation

Health education specialists can play important roles in the legislative process. They can be very active and vocal on a number of issues, such as water quality, health care reform, motorcycle safety helmets, clean air efforts, smoking restrictions, etc. The activity may take the forms of group organization to help introduce and support legislation, letter-writing campaigns, rallies, visiting and phone-in to legislators. Health education specialists may join professional organizations who will work on behalf of their membership to influence legislation. These organizations may publish position papers of given issues or hire lobbyists to educate legislators on the professions' positions.

Freedom from Lay Control

At this time in the health education and health promotion profession, there is freedom from outside control. Much of the control over health education and health promotion practitioners is exercised by peers and not consumers. Health education and health promotion research and publication is a largely peer-reviewed process. Grant applications are largely reviewed and monitored by peers.

Strength of Identity

The health education professionals will form and maintain strong identification with the profession, by committing to the life's work or calling of the profession. They will become professionally socialized and develop values, attitudes, and beliefs that support their roles as health education specialists (Siegel, 1968). The commitment to and identity with the profession may be demonstrated in the scholarly production of research and publications. This scholarly production also includes teaching. Also, many health education specialists exhibit the identity through service activities, sharing their expertise in communities, schools, and places of worship. Membership in professional organizations supports the practitioner's socialization into the profession, offering networking opportunities, employment services, opportunities to present papers, and to serve in leadership roles in the profession. Some of the professional organizations available to health education specialists are:

Society for Public Health Education (SOPHE)

Coalition of National Health Education Organizations (CNHEO)

Society of State Directors of Health, Physical Education and Recreation (SSDHPER)

Association of State and Territorial Directors of Health Promotion and Public Health Education (ASTDHPPHE)

American Association for Health Education (AAHE)

American Public Health Association (APHA)

American College Health Association (ACHA)

International Union for Health Promotion and Education (IUHPE)

Association for Worksite Health Promotion (AWHP)

Eta Sigma Gamma (ESA)

National Wellness Association (NWA)

Canadian Public Health Association (CPHA)

Areas of Health Education Responsibilities in the Profession

The professional role and practice of the health education specialist are defined by the responsibilities, competencies, and sub-competencies for entry-level health educators first described in the *Framework for the Development of Competency-Based Curricula for Entry Level Health Educators* (National Task Force on the Preparation and Practice of Health Educators, 1985). These responsibilities and competencies were applicable to all health education specialists regardless of degree held, years of experience or practice setting. The Health Educator Job Analysis 2010 (HEJA-2010) was published in 2010 and was responsible for validating the practice of advanced and entry-level health educators, developing the materials for the CHES and MCHES exams, reporting changes in the practice of health education since 2005, and informing professionals about continuing education (AAHE, NCHEC, & SOPHE, 2010). Additionally, HEJA-2010 validated the seven major responsibilities, 34 competencies, and 162 sub-competencies which specify the scope of practice for health educators (AAHE, NCHEC, & SOPHE, 2010). The seven areas of responsibility are a comprehensive set of competencies and sub-competencies which define the role of the health education specialist.

Presented here are the HEJA-2010 seven areas of responsibility with brief descriptions. For the complete listing of the responsibilities, competencies, and sub-competencies, see Appendix B.

Responsibility 1: Assess Needs, Assets, and Capacity for Health Education

The first responsibility for health educators involves assessing needs, assets, and capacity for health education/promotion. This responsibility of assessment provides the foundation for health education program planning and is a key step in the planning process. A needs assessment is defined as "a process that helps program planners determine what health problems might exist in any given group of people, what assets are available in the community to address the health problems, and the overall

Reprinted by permission of The National Commission for Health Education Credentialing, Inc., Society for Public Health Education (SOPHE), and American Association for Health Education (AAHE).

capacity of the community to address the health issues" (McKenzie, et. al., 2009). Other terms used to describe this process are community diagnosis, community analysis and community assessment.

Competency 1.1 Plan Assessment Process

Competency 1.2 Access Existing Information and Data Related to Health

Competency 1.3 Collect Quantitative and/or Qualitative Data Related to Health

Competency 1.4 Examine Relationships Among Behavioral, Environmental, and Genetic Factors That Enhance or Compromise Health

Competency 1.5 Examine Factors That Influence the Learning Process

Competency 1.6 Examine Factors That Enhance or Compromise the Process of Health Education

Competency 1.7 Infer Needs for Health Education Based on Assessment Findings

Responsibility II: Plan Health Education

Successful health education interventions involve planning that actually begins with the assessment and its findings, the review of the determined health needs, definition of the problem or issue, a hypothesis on how the problem will be solved, the selection of the theoretical framework, and the involvement of the target population. The stakeholders who are the community leaders, representatives from community organizations, resource providers, and representatives of the population are identified during the assessment process. They are then recruited to participate in the planning of the program with the health education specialist. The health education specialist with the support of the planning group will develop goals and measurable objectives. The goals and the measurable objectives will guide the planners in developing the appropriate intervention, and selecting appropriate strategies, methods, and activities.

Competency 2.1 Involve Priority Populations and Other Stakeholders in the Planning Process

Competency 2.2 Develop Goals and Objectives

Competency 2.3 Select or Design Strategies and Interventions

Competency 2.4 Develop a Scope and Sequence for the Delivery of Health Education

Competency 2.5 Address Factors That Affect Implementation

Reprinted by permission of The National Commission for Health Education Credentialing, Inc., Society for Public Health Education (SOPHE), and American Association for Health Education (AAHE).

Responsibility III: Implement Health Education

After the initial plan is developed it is time to implement the program. This means that it is time to take the plan off the drawing board and put it into action. However, even the implementation of the health education intervention must be planned to be sure that all aspects of the plan are followed according to the schedule for implementation. This is often an exciting period for the health education specialist and the planning team. To assure success in the implementation phase the health education specialist must know and understand the target population receiving the intervention before the implementation. Appropriate trained staff, strategies, methods, and materials must be utilized in the most effective and efficient way to avoid waste of limited resources. The health education specialist continues to monitor the intervention throughout its implementation to be sure that all goes as planned. Before, during, and after the implementation of the intervention, all activities and the services rendered to the program participants must be ethical, according to the Code of Ethics for health education specialists (Appendix A).

Competency 3.1 Implement a Plan of Action

Competency 3.2 Monitor Implementation of Health Education

Competency 3.3 Train Individuals Involved in Implementation of Health Education

Responsibility IV: Conduct Evaluation and Research Related to Health Education

The only way to know if health education is successful is through evaluation. The evaluation of an intervention must be planned to assure accurate measurements of the interventions components, the interventions impact for the subjects and the outcomes related to health behaviors, health status, and lifestyle changes. Effective evaluation will help to determine if resources were appropriately used in a cost effective manner. A variety of methods can be used for evaluation; they can be simple or complicated; quantitative or qualitative. The evaluation will require the health education specialists to have skills in data collection, data analysis, and interpretation of the results that may improve future health education efforts.

Competency 4.1 Develop Evaluation/Research Plan

Competency 4.2 Design Instruments to Collect

Competency 4.3 Collect and Analyze Evaluation/Research Data

Competency 4.4 Interpret Results of the Evaluation/Research

Competency 4.5 Apply Findings From Evaluation/Research

Reprinted by permission of The National Commission for Health Education Credentialing, Inc., Society for Public Health Education (SOPHE), and American Association for Health Education (AAHE).

Responsibility V: Administer and Manage Health Education

The success of a health education intervention is dependent on effective administration, management, and coordination. Health education specialists must be skilled in encouraging cooperation among personnel within programs and across programs. Often health education specialists who gain important experience in managing and administering health education programs become program managers or staff supervisors. These administrative and management responsibilities can be performed by exceptional entry level health education specialists, but they are usually assigned to those at more advanced levels of practice.

Competency 5.1 Manage Fiscal Resources

Competency 5.2 Obtain Acceptance and Support for Programs

Competency 5.3 Demonstrate Leadership

Competency 5.4 Manage Human Resources

Competency 5.5 Facilitate Partnerships in Support of Health Education

Responsibility VI: Serve as a Health Education Resource Person

With so many people, groups and organizations interested in improving their health, it is not unusual for health education specialists to get many requests for health information, counseling or consulting. Health education specialists are often called upon to serve as resource persons. If schools do not have a health educator on staff, the community or public health educator may be called on to provide teaching or other services to the schools. Parents may seek the advice or help of a health education specialist to address concerns that they have for their children. Health education specialists must be able to not only provide accurate health information, but must be able to deliver it in a professional manner, provide counseling services and consultative services as a resource person. Some health education specialists decide to focus their careers as resource persons.

Competency 6.1 Obtain and Disseminate Health-Related Information

Competency 6.2 Provide Training

Competency 6.3 Serve as a Health Education Consultant

Reprinted by permission of The National Commission for Health Education Credentialing, Inc., Society for Public Health Education (SOPHE), and American Association for Health Education (AAHE).

Responsibility VII: Communicate and Advocate for Health and Health Education

The very nature and mission of the health education specialist mean that he or she must be able to communicate and interact with various people. Effective and appropriate communication must be conducted with patient populations, community leaders and representatives, legislators, government representatives and administrators, other health professionals, consumers, students, employers, employees, and other health educators. The health education specialist must be adept at translating difficult scientific concepts to lay audiences enabling them to improve their health. Health educators may have more time to actually work with an individual or group until they are able to grasp important concepts. They also will have a ready arsenal of methods and materials that can be used to help clients or others grasp important concepts necessary for changing health behaviors. The health education specialist is called on to be an advocate for legislation, policies and resources that will improve the health of their constituents.

Competency 7.1 Assess and Prioritize Health Information and Advocacy Needs

Competency 7.2 Identify and Develop a Variety of Communication Strategies, Methods, and Techniques

Competency 7.3 Deliver Messages Using a Variety of Strategies, Methods, and Techniques

Competency 7.4 Engage in Health Education Advocacy

Competency 7.5 Influence Policy to Promote Health

Competency 7.6 Promote the Health Education Profession

Reprinted by permission of The National Commission for Health Education Credentialing, Inc., Society for Public Health Education (SOPHE), and American Association for Health Education (AAHE).

References

American Association for Health Education. 2008. *2008 NCATE Health Education Teacher Preparation Standards.* Retrieved on May 5, 2013.

Balog, J. E., J. H. Shireffs, R. D. Gutierrez, and L. F. Balog. 1985. "Ethics and the Field of Health Education." *The Eta Sigma Gamma Monograph Series* 4 (1): 65–110.

Butler, J. T. 2001. *Principles of Health Education and Health Promotion.* Belmont, CA: Wadsworth/Thomson Learning.

Cottrell, R. R., J. T. Girvan, and J. F. McKenzie. 2012. *Principles and Foundations of Health Promotion and Education.* Boston: Benjamin Cummings.

Council on Education in Public Health. 2012. *U.S. Schools of Public Health and Graduate Public Health Programs Accredited by the Council on Education in Public Health.* Retrieved on May 5, 2013, from http://ceph.org/.

National Commission for Health Education Credentialing, Inc. (NCHEC), Society for Public Health Education (SOPHE), American Association for Health Education (AAHE). (2010a). *A Competency-based Framework for Health Education Specialists–2010.* Retrieved on May 4, 2013, from http://www.nchec.org/credentialing/responsibilities.

National Task Force on the Preparation and Practice of Health Educators. (1985). *Framework for the Development of Competency-based Curricula for Entry Level Health Educators.* New York: National Commission for Health Education Credentialing, Inc.

Siegel, H. 1968. "Professional Socialization in Two Baccalaureate Programs." *Nursing Research* 17 (5): 403–7.

Thiroux, J. P. 1995. *Ethics: Theory and Practice,* 5th ed. Englewood Cliffs, NJ: Prentice-Hall.

Thomasma, D. C. 1979. "Human Values and Ethics: Professional Responsibility." *The Journal of the American Dietetic Association* 75 (5): 533–6.

Tschudin, V. 2003. *Ethics in Nursing: The Caring Relationship,* 3rd ed. Edinburgh, Scotland: Butterworth Heinemann.

Chapter 5

The Settings for Health Education and Health Promotion Practice

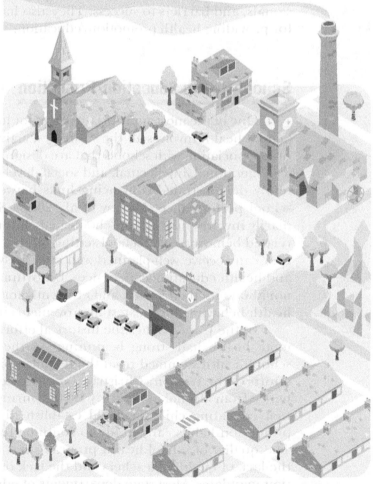

© John M. Fischer, 2013. Used under license from Shutterstock, Inc.

Health education professionals are specially trained to help individuals and communities reduce their health risks and increase the likelihood of living long, productive lives. Health education specialists perform their responsibilities in a variety of settings. The responsibilities and the health education process are generally the same, but the clientele, the needs, will vary according to the settings in which they serve. The fact that health education specialists practice in multiple settings allows the very important health education and health promotion services to be available to the greatest number of people with their many health challenges. This also means that the health education specialists will apply their competencies and will develop new competencies that meet the specific professional job descriptions for the specific settings and employers. Most professional preparation programs in health education/promotion usually prepare students for employment in schools, health care centers/hospitals, public/community health agencies, worksites/business, colleges/university, the military, international organizations, and the faith community. According to the Bureau of Labor, over 63,400 health education specialists were employed in the United States in 2010 (Bureau of Labor Statistics, 2012). All of these settings have their own unique needs, requirements for professionals, and barriers to success. They also have their own distinct reasons for providing health promotion/education.

School Health Education/Promotion

One of the most appropriate places for health education is the school. School health involves all the strategies, activities, and services offered by or in association with schools that are designed to promote students' physical, emotional, intellectual, and social development. Research has consistently demonstrated convincing links between good health and strong school performance (Murray et al., 2007). School health education primarily involves instructing school-aged children about health and health-related behaviors. The school setting offers a captive audience of students who can receive well-planned and effectively delivered health education and health education experiences. Unfortunately, these opportunities are not always used effectively and efficiently for greatest success in changing health behaviors for greatest improvements in health.

In the United States the historical efforts to control disease and promote health had strong beginnings in the schools. Initial impetus for school health stemmed from the terrible epidemics of the 1800s and the efforts of the Women's Christian Temperance Movement to promote abstinence from alcohol in the early 1900s. During this period leaders thought that educating children could establish disease prevention and health promotion habits early in life to continue throughout life (Butler, 2001). The quality of school health programs has often been compromised by the lack of qualified teachers and the lack of strict enforcement of education mandates. Most state departments of education do have mandates or regulations requiring health education in the school curricula for kindergarten through the 12th grade.

Today, school-based health education provides the opportunities to significantly influence positive health-related change in the lives of youth and address health and education goals through Coordinated School Health Programs (CSHP). The CSHP is currently known as the Coordinated School Health (CSH). The CSH puts both student health and well-being along with academic achievement at the center of its mission (Telljohann et al., 2012). The following are the components of CSH.

- Comprehensive school health instruction, built around the National Health Education Standards

- School health services

- Healthy school environment

- Nutrition services

- Community and family involvement

- Physical education

- School psychological, counseling/guidance, and social services

- Health education and promotion programs for faculty and staff

When properly implemented, CSH promotes wellness and motivation for health maintenance and improvement among students, their families, and the school staff because of the following features: CSH offers educational opportunities for the family and community, offers leadership and coordination through an effective management system, and provides planned ongoing in-service programs (Telljohann et al., 2012). The CSH requires continual assessment and evaluation for continuing relevance and success. All schools have implemented some components of the CSH, but it is rare when all eight components have been fully developed. Many school districts are concerned with financial challenges and are concerned about the cost of such efforts, but high quality school health education is cost effective when it is carefully planned and is based upon a realistic assessment of pupil needs, interests, and capabilities.

The goal of health education and health promotion in schools is to help students adopt and maintain healthy behaviors that they will apply throughout life. The school health education specialists must be well trained and prepared to deliver comprehensive standards-based curriculum. Most school districts offer health education, and thus need health teachers. However, some school districts hire individuals not specifically trained in health education. This can significantly reduce or eliminate the intent, effectiveness, and impact of the school health education goals and programming. Those health education specialists who want to be hired into school districts may perform substitute teaching, coaching, and volunteering in the schools to increase their chances for employment. While teaching is the primary function of the school health educator, school health education specialists are encouraged to take leadership roles in advocating for and developing school health policies. These policies may include food service options, safety measures, violence and suicide prevention, staff wellness, and community advisory committees.

Public/Community Health Education/Promotion

There is often confusion over the terms public health education/promotion or community health education/promotion. Health education specialists in both of these areas have similar skill sets, meet the competencies of the National Commission for Health Education Credentialing, and compete for similar jobs. The differences in public health and community health lie in their sources of funding and areas of focus. Public health programs are usually government funded through taxation that support initiatives and mandates serving individuals, local communities, states, and the nation in health education and health promotion. Community health programs are largely supported by community and voluntary health agencies that are funded by citizen donations, grants, and endowments. The health education specialists in both of these areas focus on the health of the community recognizing the health of the community is directly linked to the health of the community members. Voluntary health agencies and public health agencies are the most likely sources of employment for community health education specialists.

Community health agencies or voluntary health agencies play a larger role in the United States than in most other countries. Some examples of such agencies and organizations are the American Heart Association, the American Diabetes Association, the United Way, the American Cancer Society, etc. Voluntary health agencies are created to deal with health needs not met by governmental agencies. Much of their funding is used to provide services and support research for their areas of interests. Health education specialists are hired to plan, implement, and evaluate the education component of the agency's programs. Administratively, health education specialists may be involved in such duties as coordinating volunteers, budgeting, fund-raising, and serving as liaisons to other agencies and groups.

Public health education specialists are found in departments of public health that are formed to coordinate and provide health services to communities as mandated by laws and governmental directives. Health departments may be organized by the city, county, state, or federal government. In these departments, health education specialists serve in a variety of roles that will include assessment of populations, program planning, implementation, evaluation, grant writing and program administration. They will deliver direct services to the community and it's members through teaching, training, counseling, and consulting. They often serve as liaisons to other agencies and groups, building coalitions to address community health challenges. In public health, health education specialists perform their duties with diverse populations, addressing the needs of and partnering with people of various income levels, ages, races and ethnicities, cultures, genders, and political views. Within the public health environment they will work in concert with other health professionals to solve community health problems.

Worksite Health Education/Promotion

Worksite health promotion is defined as a combination of educational, organizational, and environmental activities designed to improve the health and safety of employees and their families (Cottrell et. al., 2012). Many businesses and organizations offer health care insurance to their workers. The costs of employee health benefits have increased for employers. The concerns for cost containment and the well-being of their employees have generated greater interests in the development and implementation of worksite wellness programs. These programs offer health promotion services for employees and their family members, often reducing the health care costs and health problems which are largely the result of behavioral issues. Health promotion programs at worksites differ greatly from site to site, because of differences in the businesses' goals, and types of employees. The proportion of employers providing worksite health promotion programs has increased over the years, with some kind of programming offered in over 80% of worksites with 50 or more employees, and almost all large employers with more than 750 employees (Cottrell et. al., 2012).

Health education specialists must be able to market a health promotion program to the management of a company, because the administrators are always concerned about getting the best return on their investments. The management of companies is most concerned about improving the health of their employees to reduce absenteeism, address an aging workforce, eliminate worksite injuries, reduce health insurance premiums, and to increase retention of employees, their job satisfaction and to improve morale. Companies are also interested in being perceived as innovators for their respective industries and among their employees. Worksite wellness programs that are successful, present the employers in a very positive light for the employees, their families and the community.

Health education specialists in worksite wellness are likely to have competencies that allow them to fulfill all of the health education responsibilities (assessment, planning, implementing, and evaluating programs and services), as well as expertise in physical fitness, diet and nutrition, stress management, etc. that are common areas of interest for employees. Working in worksite wellness programs, health education specialists will have duties that include the use of media in creating bulletin boards, newsletters, coordinating annual health fairs, conducting companywide screenings, and initiating and monitoring flu shot programs.

Passage of the Patient Protection and Affordable Care Act is expected to bring about significant changes for worksite health promotion in the form of increased opportunities to establish wellness programs and offer employee rewards in the form of insurance premium discounts. However, the legislation is presenting major challenges for employers who must support changes financially, resulting in the reduction in workforce for some companies.

Medical and Health Care Settings

Many positions exists for health education specialists in medical clinics, hospitals, community health care centers, and managed care organizations. Health education specialists in the medical care field serve as administrators, directors, managers, and coordinators, supporting and consulting on health education programs and services. Providing patient education is another way health education specialists have been used in a health care setting.

Health education specialists may provide worksite wellness programs and services to employees of the health care facilities. Because health insurance companies do not typically reimburse for patient education services; the hospitals, clinics, and physicians rarely offer health promotion and education services to their patients. HMOs have been most receptive to hiring health education specialists. Current changes in the medical care system, increased emphases on cost-cutting measures, and movement toward managed care should bring greater employment opportunities for health education specialists within the health care settings. In the various health care settings, health education specialist can expect to have expertise in grant writing, one-on-one or group patient education services, publicity, public relations, and employee wellness activities as some of the responsibilities beyond planning, implementing, and evaluating services and programs.

Health Education/Promotion in Colleges and Universities

The number and quality of health promotion programs have greatly increased on the campuses of universities and colleges. Many of these wellness centers are like health care centers with doctors and nurses on staff to care for minor health problems. However, the missions of most of these centers are to support the growth and development of students, to prevent diseases and to promote health among students and the university community. These wellness centers also support health promotion services for faculty and staff which is more like the functions of worksite health centers. Health education specialists are employed by university health services or wellness centers. They may be health education professionals with undergraduate degrees, but usually the master's degree in health education is preferred. If this professional is considered a member of the academic faculty, a doctoral degree and prior experience are usually required with major responsibilities for teaching, community and professional service, and scholarly research.

Health education specialists will have major responsibility for planning, implementing, and evaluating health promotion and education programs for program participants, which will include students, faculty, and staff. Other duties will include developing health education materials, maintaining a resource library, one-on-one counseling with students, developing and coordinating a peer education program, speaking to student groups, and planning special events.

International Opportunities

A variety of positions exists in international organizations for professionals with health education training. Many positions exist to help residents in developing countries to improve their health and the quality of their lives. Often these positions require special dedication due to unusual and sometimes difficult, working or living conditions. Working in international situations requires knowledge of and sensitivities to indigenous cultures. Working internationally requires examination of different health conditions, social conditions and political environments. Health education specialists must be willing to try culturally appropriate interventions to encourage the communities' participation in the planning and implementation process and to achieve successful behavior changes.

The Military

Our government has always been committed to the health of our armed forces. A healthy military provides greater safety and protection for the citizens of this country. The nutritional status and physical fitness have always been of great interests. The military then provides an important setting for health education and health promotion for the military forces and their families. The military focus in health promotion is to optimize the total effectiveness and efficiency of the armed forces. The military is also concerned about cost containment related to treating diseases, injuries, and disabilities. Health promotion helps to reduce those costs.

Health education and health promotion in the military is similar to the work that is performed in worksite wellness programs. Many of the functions and responsibilities of the health education specialists in the military will be similar to those of the health education specialists in worksite wellness programs. These specialists in the military may come from the military health professionals or they may be civilians hired to perform health education services for the military. The professional preparation and responsibilities are the same as the other health education specialists in diverse community and health care services.

The Faith Community

Formal communities of faith are important and significant settings for health education and health promotion. Early in the history of human beings there existed strong relationships between peoples' faith and religious practices and their health. Those same connections exist today among many of our citizens and communities. It appears that these communities of believers will again be important to improving the health and quality of life of these citizens.

The faith community itself is mobilizing and focusing on health promotion interventions among their congregants and the communities. Significant research findings show that active faith or religiosity improves immunity to communicable diseases, reduces the incidence of many chronic diseases, extends the survival rate of surgery patients, improves social interaction, reduces stress and anxiety, and generally makes people healthier and happier (Breckon et. al., 1998; Butler, 2001). Anyone seeking employment in faith-based organizations should research the beliefs and goals of such organizations thoroughly to avoid misunderstandings and conflicts. Besides the competencies and responsibilities of the professional health educator, an interfaith organization described six characteristics of health education specialists who would serve faith communities (Interfaith Health Program, 1997):

- The ability to listen to the community;

- The possession of natural leadership ability;

- Respected by the community;

- Actively participate in the health education process with the community;

- Demonstration of honest concern for the health and wellness of others;

- Understanding that health goes beyond just medicine and incorporates the spiritual well-being in the total health of individuals.

Non-Traditional Health Education/Promotion Positions

The professional trained in the responsibilities and competencies for health education will find career potential in a number of less traditional fields. There are many opportunities available to health education specialists who are committed to informing, teaching and training people in health promotion and health education in nontraditional fields. Sales positions related to health, such as pharmacy sales, fitness equipment sales, and sales of health-related textbooks offer great opportunities for health education specialists. Journalism and broadcasting provide career opportunities for health or medical reporters and for authors of health articles in newspaper, magazines, or web-based services. The criminal justice and mental health systems can provide careers working as a teacher, drug educator, sexuality educator, or counselor.

References

American School Health Association. 2013. *What is School Health?* Retrieved May 22, 2013, from http://www.ashaweb.org/i4a/pages/index.cfm?pageid=3278.

Association of Schools of Public Health. 2013. Careers in Public Health. Retrieved May 12, 2013 from http://www.whatispublichealth.org/careers/index.html.

Breckon, J., J. R. Harvey, and R. B. Lancaster. 1998. *Community Health Education: Settings, Roles, Skills for the 21st Century.* Gaithersburg, MD: Aspen Publishers.

Bureau of Labor Statistics, US Department of Labor, *Occupational Outlook Handbook, 2012-13 Edition*, Health Educators. Retrieved on June 01, 2013 from http://www.bls.gov/ooh/community-and-social-service/health-educators.htm.

Butler, J. T. 2001. *Principles of Health Education and Health Promotion.* Belmont, CA: Wadsworth/Thomson Learning.

Centers for Disease Control and Prevention (CDC). 2013. *Career Opportunities in Global Health.* Retrieved April 10, 2013, from http://www.cdc.gov/globalhealth/employment/pdf/Global%20Health%20recruitment%20 brochure(links).pdf.

Cottrell, R. R., J. T. Girvan, and J. F. McKenzie. 2012. *Principles and Foundations of Health Promotion and Education.* Boston: Benjamin Cummings.

Daitz, S. J. 2007. "Health Education Careers at Nonprofit Voluntary Health Agencies." *Health Education Monograph* 24 (1): 4–6.

Interfaith Health Program, The Carter Center. 1997. *Starting Point: Empowering Communities to Improve Health—A Manual for Training Health Promoters in Congregational Coalitions.* Atlanta, GA.

Murray, N., B. Low, A. Cross, and S. Davis. 2007. "Coordinated School Health Programs and Academic Achievement: A Systematic Review of the Literature." *Journal of School Health* 77 (9): 589–600.

National Task Force on the Preparation and Practice of Health Educators. 1985. *Framework for the Development of Competency-Based Curricula for Entry Level Health Educators.* New York: National Commission for Health Education Credentialing, Inc.

National Task Force on the Preparation and Practice of Health Educators. 2013. *Health Education Profession.* Retrieved on April 10, 2013 from http://www.nchec.org/credentialing/profession/.

Telljohann, Susan K., C. W. Symons, B. Pateman, D. M. Seabert. 2012. *Health Education: Elementary and Middle School Applications*, 7th edition. New York: McGraw-Hill Companies, Inc.

Totzkay-Sitar, C., and S. Cornett. 2007. "Health Education Options in Health and Medical Care." *The Health Education Monograph* 24 (1): 7–10.

Chapter 6

Changing Health Behaviors: An Overview

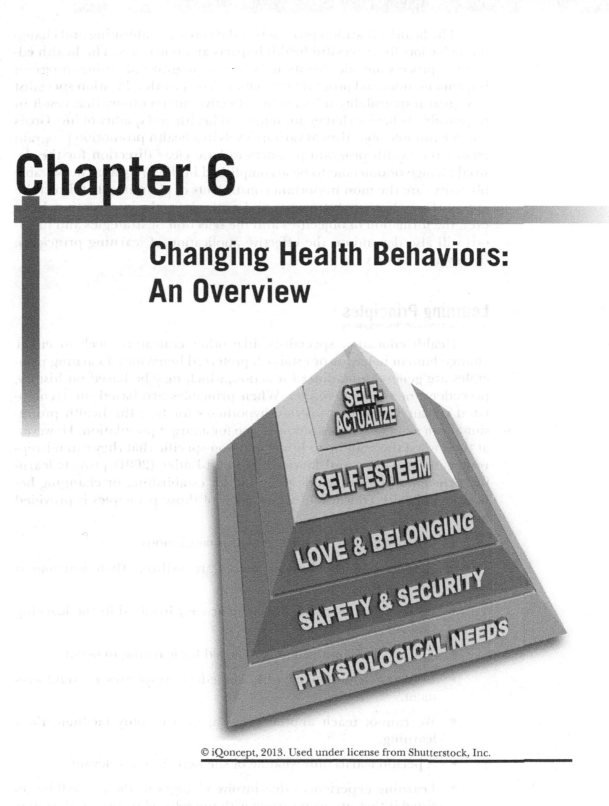

© iQoncept, 2013. Used under license from Shutterstock, Inc.

The health education process is at the core of establishing and changing behaviors for successful health impacts and outcomes. The health education process includes needs assessments, program planning, program implementation, and program evaluation. The health education specialist has great responsibility in planning effective interventions that result in responsible behavior change for improved health and quality of life. Goals and measurable objectives at various levels in a health promotion program enable the health program planners to have clear direction for the desired change or outcome to be accomplished in the program. Measurable objectives are the most important constituents of planning that direct the appropriate selection of strategies and methods for the intervention. However, the formation of objectives and the selection of strategies and methods will also depend on the effective application of learning principles, theory, and models.

Learning Principles

Health education specialists, like other educators, seek to either change human behavior or establish preferred behaviors. Learning principles are general guidelines for action, which may be based on history, precedent, or research results. When principles are based on accumulated research, they can provide hypotheses for how the health professional can achieve the desired outcome for a target population. However, at their worst they can be so broad and non-specific that they can misrepresent reality. Green and Lewis (1986) and Butler (2001) provide learning principles that can guide planning for establishing or changing behaviors in health education. An overview of those principles is provided here:

- Learning is not a single event, it is continuous.

- If several of the human senses are utilized then learning is facilitated.

- People learn by doing, by being actively involved in the learning process.

- The learner's motivation is required for learning to occur.

- Learning is enhanced with immediate responses or reinforcement.

- We cannot teach another person, we can only facilitate their learning.

- A person learns only what he or she perceives as relevant.

- Learning experiences that involve changes in the self will be resisted if they are inconsistent with the self; relaxation of the self is required so that learning can be facilitated.

Gilbert et. al., (2011) also provide some basic educational principles that can help planners choose appropriate methods and sequence methods for interventions:

- Repetition is usually required for learning to occur. At least three exposures to the content are recommended.

- Learning is an active process involving dynamic interaction of the learner and the content being learned.

- Learning usually advances from the simple to the complex, from the known to the unknown and from the concrete to the abstract.

- Transfer learning is not automatic; so teaching should focus on transfer which is the ability to apply prior knowledge or skills to new situations.

- Behaviors and skills that are being taught must be practiced.

- Periods of practice with intermittent periods of rest result in more efficient learning.

Sometimes broad and non-specific principles may generate multiple interpretations and are unreliable. Theory goes beyond principle (Glanz, 1997).

Theories and Models in Health Education and Health Promotion

Health promotion and health education planning have foundations based in a multidisciplinary field of practice. Health promotion planning is most likely to be effective and successful when the process and plan is theory-based and theory-driven. The foundations of health promotion have evolved from various fields of practice such as biological, sociological, behavioral and health science disciplines. These disciplines, especially the social and behavioral sciences offer foundational theories and models that can guide the health education specialists in trying to explain existing human behavior, predict future behavior, and to plan interventions to bring about desired changes in health behavior and health status for individuals and communities. These theories are meaningful in health education and health promotion when accompanied by the specialists' strong foundations in biological sciences, epidemiology, biostatistics, and cultural competence.

Helping individuals, families, and communities establish responsible health behaviors is the central concern of health promotion and health education. Health behaviors are the actions of individuals, groups, organizations, and communities, and their associated determinants, correlates and consequences, i.e., social change, policy development and implementation, and enhanced quality of life (Glanz et. al., 1997). Theories provide tools to the health education specialist to use in examining health problems and in planning interventions to solve health problems.

Theory Defined

Glanz et. al., (1997) state that "a theory is a set of interrelated concepts, definitions, and propositions that presents a systematic view of events or situations by specifying relations among variables in order to explain and predict the events of the situations." A theory offers a general and simplified explanation of "why people act or do not act to maintain and/or promote the health of themselves, their families, organizations, and communities (Cottrell et. al., 2012, p. 100)." Theories have three important characteristics. They have generality, so that they can be applied broadly to a variety of health issues. Secondly, they are testable. Credible theory is supported by a strong research foundation that tests the theory in real health issues and applications. Thirdly, theories are abstract. According to Blalock (1969), theory does not represent a real system in the social sciences nor in health promotion and education; it only approximates reality. It is important to remember that theory deals with the ideal more than with the real.

Like empty coffee cups, theories have shapes and boundaries, but nothing inside. They become useful when filled with practical topics, goals, and problems (Glanz and Rimer, 2005).

Theories can be classified as explanatory theories or theories of the problem, and change theories or theories of action (Sharma & Romas, 2012). Explanatory theory describes the reasons for why a problem exists, guiding the health education specialists' search for factors that contribute to a problem and that can be targeted for change. Examples of explanatory theories include the Health Belief Model and the Theory of Planned Behavior. Change theory guides the health education specialists in developing meaningful health interventions for defined health problems. It presents the concepts that can be translated into interventions, methods, and strategies, and offers a basis for program evaluation. Change theory helps program planners to be explicit about their assumptions for why a program will work. Two examples of change theories include Community Organization and Diffusion of Innovations.

While only a limited number of theories are presented in this textbook, theories, and models from a variety of disciplines explain problems, explain behaviors, and suggest ways to achieve behavioral change. A theoretical foundation provides researchers and program planners with a perspective from which to organize knowledge and to interpret factors and events. By telling the program planner the what, how, when, and why of a given health issue, theories can help guide program development in health education and health promotion. The "what" tells the planner the elements that should be considered as the targets for the intervention. The "why" informs the planners about the processes by which changes occur in the target variables. The "when" tells the planner about the timing and sequencing of planned interventions in order to achieve maximum effects. The "how" describes the methods and activities the planner will use to focus interventions; it includes the specific means of inducing changes in the explanatory variables. (Glanz, Lewis, & Rimer, 1990)

Models

Models are similar to theories when the theories are in the early development. Models are presented without the empirical evidence that is required for a theory. They may actually draw on a number of theories to help understand a particular problem in a certain setting or context. They are not as specified as theory. Models can be eclectic in the choices of theories that are used in them. Models can be used for guidance in the planning process. Many models are utilized to inform the program planning process, such as, PRECEDE-PROCEED (Green and Kreuter, 2005), social marketing, ecological planning approaches (Green et. al., 1994; Glanz et. al., 2005). In these cases, the models can serve as the vehicles by which the theories are applied. As previously stated, an example of a model used extensively for guidance in program planning is the PRECEDE-PROCEED (Green and Kreuter, 2005). This model provides guidance for planning at the macro level, helping health education planners identify the behaviors that must be targeted, what resources are available to use, how to mobilize the community, etc. Theories can provide guidance at the micro level, helping to identify the attitudes to change for health behavior change, the activities that are best for the targeted audience, which methods to employ, etc. (Sharma, 2012). There are models that have been thoroughly tested and are considered theories, but still have the word "model" in their names. The Health Belief Model and the Transtheoretical Model are examples of models that have undergone significant testing and have generated significant research findings supporting their use in program planning.

Theory Components

The critical components of a theory are constructs, concepts, variables, and constants. See Figure 6.1. Constructs are the building blocks of

Figure 6.1 Conceptual representation of a theory

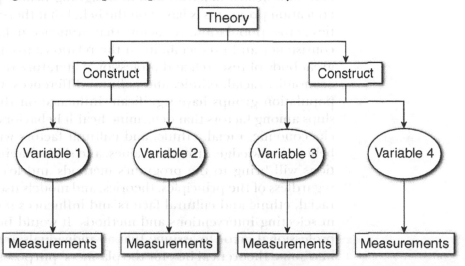

a theory and represent the primary elements and major components of a theory. Constructs are described as latent variables that lack empiricism; which means they cannot be observed through taste, touch, vision, smell, or hearing. Constructs organize and combine concepts or variables into one group or under one subheading in a theory. Constructs are specific and can be used only within the context of a given theory. Constructs are concepts and variables that have been developed or adopted for use in a particular theory (Kerlinger, 1986). Cornish (1980) described a concept as a generalized idea, a mental map or an image of some phenomena. A group of concepts under a given construct must have cohesion that is logical and real (Ledlow and Coppola, 2012). Actually concepts are variables or constants in a theory. Variables are defined as the empirical counterparts or the operational forms of constructs; meaning that they can be measured or observed by the senses (Green and Lewis, 1986; Glanz et. al., 1997). They are universally described and recognized. Variables can be measured and the measurements can vary or change. An example would be "weight." The variables direct how constructs in a given situation are to be measured. According to Glanz and Rimer (2005), variables should be matched to constructs when determining what should be measured in the evaluation of a theory-driven program.

Constants are concepts that do not vary or change. Sex can be a constant in some situations. In a program or research on the course of pregnancy, the sex of all participants would be female, a constant. However, in a program or research on heart disease, sex would be a variable that would identify participants as male or female.

The success of a program in health education and health promotion will depend on the health educators' uses of the most appropriate theories, models, and related practice strategies for a given health issue. Differing theories apply to different units of practice: individuals, groups, organizations, and communities. The selection of the theory begins with the problem definition, the hypothesis, the goal, the unit of practice, and the context of the practitioner's activities.

The use of theory in explaining, understanding, and predicting human and health behavior and in designing health promotion and health education programs is based on the belief that there are some commonalities across populations in factors that influence behavior and that there is consistency and predictability in the relationships among these factors. A great body of research and professional literature demonstrates that socioeconomic, racial, ethnic, and cultural differences among individuals and population groups have significant influence on the theoretical relationships among factors that determine health behaviors and health status. Socioeconomic, racial, ethnic, and cultural factors will often represent the beliefs, knowledge, attitudes, values, and skills that individuals and populations will bring to the program's methods and learning experiences. So regardless of the principles, theories, and models used, the socioeconomic, racial, ethnic and cultural factors and influences must also be considered in selecting interventions and methods. It would be a fatal program and professional error to assume that all individuals are the same and will fit into some theoretical box for the planners' purposes.

Learning and Behavior

Behavioral change will occur through developmental maturation, through learning or through both processes. Developmental maturation is the process manifested as an individual grows to fulfill his/her genetic human blueprint. Learning brings about changed behavior through experiences, insights, and perceptions. The health education specialist must be knowledgeable about both processes in helping individuals to achieve improved health outcomes. This chapter focuses on learning for behavior change and the theories that assist the professional in explaining and supporting behavioral change for improved health.

Generally, the professional literature supports that learning is more than an accumulation of knowledge. Learning is defined as a change in knowledge, skills, beliefs, attitudes, values, and behavior as a result of experience. Learning is required for survival and success. It influences decision-making about a wide range of health behaviors. However, learning is not the only influence on behavior. There are those factors that require the individual and/or communities to balance influences on their behavior: influences from personal preferences, family, friends, media, school, work, religion, culture, ethnicity, etc. These will be addressed in the discussion on the social ecological model.

Learning for behavior change involves more than the accumulation of knowledge or the collection of information. Learning actually occurs in three domains: cognitive domain, affective domain, and the psychomotor domain. The cognitive domain involves acquiring knowledge and information on an intellectual level, developing relationships with facts, truth, and principles. In health education the goal is behavior change which requires more than cognitive learning. In the cognitive domain there are certain educational objectives that must be achieved. The *Bloom's Taxonomy of Educational Objectives* (Bloom, 1956), has been instructive for educators for many years. Bloom provides a listing of cognitive objectives with examples of the cognitive abilities required for each. The following is a sampling of these cognitive abilities for each level of cognitive development.

1. *Knowledge:* naming, defining, describing, listing, identifying, matching, selecting, reproducing, labeling
2. *Comprehension:* explaining, describing, interpreting, converting, defending, distinguishing, generalizing, estimating, paraphrasing, predicting
3. *Application:* illustrating, predicting, applying, computing, changing, discovering, modifying, using, preparing, producing, relating, solving
4. *Analysis:* analyzing, categorizing, classifying, differentiating, discriminating, distinguishing, inferring, selecting, separating
5. *Synthesis:* concluding, proposing, synthesizing, composing, compiling, creating, designing, explaining, planning, revising, summarizing
6. *Evaluating:* contrasting, comparing, evaluating, appraising, concluding, describing, explaining, justifying, summarizing, supporting

While knowledge is necessary in the learning process, it is not sufficient to promote changed behavior in health. Health education specialists know that learning must also be reflected in attitudes, beliefs, values, and skills.

The affective domain relates to emotions, feelings, and attitudes. The primary goal of health education and health promotion is for people to voluntarily undertake responsible health behaviors. That means people determine what is best for them. Their choices will be personal and individual, influenced by their feelings, emotions, and attitudes about any given health issue. To force individuals to make choices against their wishes is unethical. Therefore the health education specialist through ethical programming and support services can assist populations in rational decision-making that honor their feelings, emotions, and attitudes. Appropriately planned and delivered learning experiences and new information may result in rational changed feelings, emotions, values, and attitudes about given health issues. Rational affective domain development coupled with knowledge produces attitudes, beliefs, and values that support establishing and changing health behaviors.

The psychomotor domain involves human motor skills and coordination. This domain involves the development of behavioral patterns and skills made by choice. The choices in the psychomotor domain will depend on selecting and developing specific behaviors and skills from among several alternatives. The decision-making and skill development depends on knowledge, attitudes, beliefs, and feelings, illustrating how the cognitive and the affective domain work together to affect the psychomotor domain. In other words, people will perform behaviors to support improved health, if they have the required knowledge, the emotions, and attitudes to support their desire to perform the behaviors. The work of the health education specialist is to provide learning experiences and support that help people develop the knowledge, the attitudes, beliefs, emotions and skills to voluntarily make the decisions to behave in health-enhancing ways.

Traditionally, learning and behavior are conceptualized as S-O-R: stimuli (S) are processed by the organism (O) and then produce a response (R). Learning is the result or product of stimuli, much of which are planned educational experiences. However, most stimuli are unplanned experiences and part of everyday life, coming from many places in the organism's environment. Some stimuli are planned experiences and are actually designed to influence behavior and to create new knowledge, perceptions, attitudes, feelings, experiences, and skills. Examples of such planned experiences include advertisements, marketing campaigns, and planned educational activities.

The manner in which the organism processes the stimuli determines the responses.

Figure 6.2 Conceptualization of the stimuli, organism, and response

Stimuli (S) ⟶ Organism (O) ⟶ Response(R)

The existing knowledge, previous experience, current attitudes, and even the mood, personality, gender, and socialization of the individual influences how she or he receives and processes a stimulus. The wide variation in how individuals are influenced by stimuli is partly the product of inherent human individuality, partly the product of learning, and partly the product of environmental circumstances and ongoing individual life events. The many competing stimuli are a challenge to consistency in human behavior. So humans are not passive recipients of stimuli, but active processors of stimuli. Individual responses to specific stimuli are not always immediate or predictable and are influenced by factors associated with being human—personality, capabilities, cognitive characteristics, and situational factors (Simons-Morton et. al., 1995).

Social Ecological Model

If health education specialists are to help populations become healthier, they will have to address many factors that impact health behaviors. It is not enough to address the individual and his or her behaviors only, health education specialists must reach beyond the intrapersonal level. In the Social Ecological Model of health behavior, the dimensions of health interact with the determinants of health at five hierarchical levels of influence: intrapersonal, interpersonal, organizational, community, and societal (or public policy). The health education specialist's ability to help populations change their behavior for improved health will depend on how these various levels of influence interact and impact the individual and how the individual impacts these various systems and levels of influence. The social ecological model is part of the ever expanding multi-level theories on health behavior change and has given rise to various versions of ecological perspectives. These ecological perspectives are most useful for examining behavior theories in the context of social, environmental, and cultural factors affecting disease and health interacting with various levels of influence that impact the individual and his/her health choices and behaviors. These interactions and the levels of influence must be considered in designing health education and health promotion interventions that successfully help health promotion program participants change behavior. Secondly, the model helps the investigator to plan strategies that target these multiple levels of influence on changing health risk factors and health behaviors for the individual, groups, and communities. These levels of influence include the following descriptions, but are not limited to these. McLeroy et. al. (1988) begin with the individual, but also include all the levels with which the individual interacts.

- Intrapersonal level (Individual characteristics that influence behavior): genetics, knowledge, attitudes, beliefs, values, skills, and self-efficacy.

- Interpersonal level (Family, friends, peers): Interpersonal processes and groups that provide identity and support to the individual.

- Organizational level (Churches, other organized worship centers, stores, community organizations): Providing context, rules, regulations, policies, and structures that constrain or promote behaviors for the individual, groups, and communities.

- Community level (Social networks, Community norms, Community regulations): At the community level, greater efforts are made to create healthful environment by addressing unemployment, homelessness, poverty, housing, violence, substance abuse, sedentary lifestyle that impacts the individual and the community.

- Public policy (Local, state, federal): Policies and laws that regulate or support healthy practices/actions.

Often planners and researchers combine the levels of organizations, community, and public policy into one category or level of community.

Many of the efforts to help individuals improve their risk status have centered on changing behavior at the intrapersonal levels. These have met with varying levels of success and failure. The problem is that research with multicultural populations has shown that interventions must do more than enhance the individual's knowledge and skill sets; they must also provide trusted social support in a safe environment. Family and peer support, organizational support and relevance, community factors, and cultural relevance are indeed important determinants of health for the target populations. The ecological approach or perspective demonstrates how more than one theory may be used to address health issues that are multilevel.

Figure 6.3 Social Ecological Model

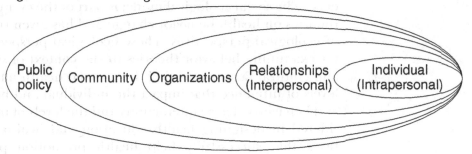

Theory at the Intrapersonal Level

Lewin's Field Theory

Kurt Lewin along with other field theorists proposed that humans, when exposed to various stimuli, will usually organize the various stimuli into meaningful wholes or gestalts, influenced by context and overall effect. They then respond to these meaningful wholes or gestalts according to their relevance to important personal needs and goals. So each individual interprets a stimulus in terms of the whole field within which the stimulus is presented and the person's perceptual context that is shaped by personal total experiences.

Field theory is important to health promoters and health educators, because it shows that each person interprets stimuli from their own personal perceptual context. In providing learning experiences, it is important not only to consider the content but also the context in which the content is delivered to the learner. This explains why the same stimulus may be highly motivating for one individual but not to another.

Lewin proposed an especially useful theory and tool called force-field analysis. Force-field analysis proposes that the forces that exist in group situations are subject to systematic analysis, and that the continuing forces within a group situation influence one another (Butler, 1997). Behavior results from two sets of forces: change or driving forces and resisting or restraining forces. With change forces, the individual or group is pressured to move toward a goal. The resisting forces will cause the individual or group to resist change. These two sets of forces work against each other constantly.

So what might be the outcomes of these sets of forces working against each other? If the total influence of the change and resisting forces is equal, there is no action by the individual or group, and no change. When the change forces are stronger than the resisting forces, individual or group behavior is changed to achieve the goal. When the resisting forces are stronger, then there is no movement toward the goal. The health education specialist can use the force field analysis to plan interventions and methods that would do the following:

- increase the influence of the driving or change forces

- reduce the influence of restraining or resisting forces

- both increase change forces and decrease the resisting forces

The health education specialist would have to identify the change forces and resisting forces acting on the target population. This information may be apparent from the needs assessment. Then the planner would determine methods for increasing the change forces and reducing the resisting forces. Focus groups, surveys and interviews in the target population can reveal valued insights that would help the planner. Most importantly, involving representatives of the target population in the planning process will certainly inform and help identify and develop the methods that will influence the change forces and the resisting forces.

Table 6.1 Smoking cessation: An example of force-field analysis

Change forces	Resisting forces
• knowledge of the health risks of smoking on the individual and his or her family • inconvenience caused by laws restricting smoking in public places • growing social isolation of smokers	• pleasure that comes from smoking • reinforcement and acceptance by their peers • difficulty of withdrawal from an addictive drug

In this situation of smoking cessation, the health education specialist may use intervention strategies and methods that would encourage family members to support a loved one's decision to stop smoking; initiate and support smoking cessation programs in the community; or increase legislation to make smoking in public more restricted. These efforts would enhance the change forces. The resisting forces can be minimized by encouraging membership in peer groups that accept and support non-smokers, and giving smokers access to the physicians who can prescribe nicotine patches to reduce withdrawal problems. Addressing both the change forces and the resisting forces will be far more effective than addressing just one set of forces.

The Health Belief Model

The Health Belief Model (HBM) was developed in the 1950's by social psychologists in the US Public Health Service as a way of explaining the overwhelming failure of people to participate in disease detection and disease prevention programs. The HBM has its basis in Lewin's decision-making model. It has been used to describe and explain several health behaviors (Janz and Becker, 1984).

HBM proposes that health-related action depends upon three categories of factors.

- the presence of sufficient motivation or health concern to make health issues relevant or prominent

- the belief of one's susceptibility or vulnerability to a serious health problem, condition, or perceived threat

- the belief that adhering to a particular health recommendation or health behavior would be beneficial in reducing the perceived threat at a personally acceptable cost. The cost relates to the perceived barriers that must be overcome to follow the recommendation (Rosenstock et. al., 1988; McKenzie and Smeltzer, 2001)

The HBM has been applied to many health behaviors to address an individual's beliefs about health and their health—specific behaviors. According to the model, the beliefs that mediate health behavior are (1) perceived susceptibility for contracting the health problem, (2) perceived severity of the health threat, (3) the perceived benefits of available and effective actions that reduce the health threat, and (4) the perceived barriers of costs or the negative aspects associated with engaging in the health behavior. Cues to action are the necessary triggers for the initiation of behavior.

According to the HBM (Rosenstock, 1974), in order for a person to take action or perform a health behavior to avoid disease or illness, he or she must believe that:

1. the individual is personally susceptible to the disease or illness

2. if the individual has the health problem, it will be severe enough to negatively affect his or her life

3. taking the recommended action or performing a recommended health behavior will have beneficial effects

4. the barriers to taking action or taking on the new behavior do not overwhelm the benefits

An HBM Application:

Carla is a health education specialist assigned to conduct classes on HIV/AIDS prevention with a group of twenty 15 and 16 year old girls. Throughout the presentation she notices restlessness and boredom. As she finishes her presentation, she questions the young ladies and finds out that they do not think her message is appropriate for them. They inform her that none of them are involved in doing drugs, and that HIV/AIDS is a problem for gay men and IV drug users.

Carla makes changes in her methods for the next session with the girls. She begins class with a video presentation on HIV/AIDS prevention that featured teenage girls and boys who had contracted HIV through heterosexual sexual intercourse. Then she introduced a young adult woman from the local speakers' bureau who had contracted HIV through heterosexual intercourse while in college. The guest speaker shared with the girls how HIV had changed her life and her dreams. That session had a very sobering effect on every girl in the class and they wanted Carla to tell them more about how to avoid the disease.

Carla was able to change methods that made her message more relevant to her target audience. She chose a video with characters and a speaker that were closer in age to the girls. The chosen methods forced the girls to heighten their perceived susceptibility to HIV/AIDS. They also began to consider the perceived benefits of changing behavior to prevent the disease. Carla understood through the Health Belief Model that helping the girls recognize their personal susceptibility, the severity of the disease, and the perceived threat of the disease would improve the likelihood of changing their behavior to personally prevent the disease in their own lives.

The Transtheoretical Model and Stages of Change

The Transtheoretical Model, or the Stages of Change, is a model that explains the stages that the majority of people seem to experience as they attempt to change health behaviors over time. Having its roots in psychotherapy, James Prochaska developed this model after he completed comparative analyses on eighteen therapy systems and a critical review of three hundred therapy outcome studies. As a result of his research Prochaska found that there were some common processes involved in behavior change. The Transtheoretical model explains that people move from precontemplation to contemplation, to preparation, to action and into maintenance (Prochaska, 1979, 1984; Prochaska and Di Clemente, 1983). These stages are precontemplation, contemplation, preparation, action, and maintenance and are defined below.

1. Precontemplation Stage: The time frame in which people are not thinking about making a change in their behavior during the next six months.

2. Contemplation Stage: The timeframe in which people become aware that a problem exists, are seriously thinking about making a change, but have not made a commitment to action.

3. Preparation Stage: People actively plan change within the next month.

4. Action Stage: People are obviously making changes in their behavior, experiences, and/or environment in order to correct a health problem.

5. Maintenance Stage: Change that starts in the action stage continues through six months after taking the obvious action that started the change in the behavior.

Besides the construct of the stages of change, the Transtheoretical Model also presents the construct for the processes of change (Prochaska et. al., 1997). The processes of change are the covert and overt activities that people use to progress through the stages of change. The health education specialist will find the construct for processes of change to be important guides for developing intervention strategies. They include for the individual:

- Consciousness raising: finding and learning new facts, ideas, and tips that support the healthy behavioral change

- Dramatic relief: experiencing the negative emotions (fear, worry, anxiety) that go along with unhealthy behavioral risks

- Self-reevaluation: realizing that the behavioral change is an important part of one's identity as a person

- Environmental re-evaluation: realizing the negative impact of the unhealthy behavior or the positive impact of the healthy behavior on one's proximal social and physical environment

- Self-liberation: making a firm commitment to change

- Helping relationships: seeking and using social support for the healthy behavioral change

- Counter-conditioning: substituting healthier alternative behaviors and cognitions for the unhealthy behaviors

- Stimulus control: removing reminders or cues to engage in the unhealthy behavior and adding cues or reminders to engage in the healthy behavior

- Social liberation: realizing that the social norms are changing in the direction of supporting the healthy behavioral change

As health education specialists help people progress through the stages of change, they must understand and apply the processes of change. The most basic principle is that different processes of change must be applied at different stages. Prochaska, DiClemente and Norcross (1992) discovered that in the early stages, people apply cognitive, affective and evaluative processes to move through the stages of change. However, in the later stages people are more involved with commitments, conditioning, contingencies, environmental controls, and support for progressing toward maintenance.

The Transtheoretical Model has been used in addressing addictive behaviors, smoking cessation, condom use, weight control and HIV prevention (McKenzie et. al., 2013). People move through behavior change at different rates. The progression through the stages of change is not linear.

The majority of people undergoing change will have relapses, which is part of the change cycle. This reminds the health education specialist that not all people are ready for change at the same time, nor do they take action for change at the same time. The model also helps the health education specialist to identify people who are ready for making changes in their health behavior, and for predicting who may be successful in changing behavior. Health education specialists can be proactive in designing programs that help individuals to become ready for change.

The Theory of Reasoned Action

The Theory of Reasoned Action developed by Fishbein and Ajzen (1975) attempts to explain volitional behaviors. It provides a way to study attitudes towards behaviors. The theory distinguishes among the constructs of attitude, belief, behavioral intention, and behavior. According to the theory, the most important determinant of behavior is a person's behavioral intention. A person's intention to engage in a particular behavior is formed by two elements:

- The person's own attitude toward performing the behavior
- The subjective norm, i.e.,
  - The person's beliefs about what significant others think the individual should do
  - How important the relevant other's opinions are to the person

The construct of subjective norm deals with the person's beliefs about what relevant others think the person should do. So a person's decision to perform a given behavior is partly dependent on what he or she believes others think he or she should do, and that the person cares about what these others think. An example of the theory of reasoned action's construct of subjective norm in health promotion is the employee who wants to enroll in a worksite weight control program, because he believes his employer wants him to do so.

The Theory of Planned Behavior

Theory of reasoned action is most effective in "dealing with purely volitional behaviors, but complications are encountered when the theory is applied to behaviors that are not fully under volitional control (McKenzie and Smeltzer, 1997)." Even when an individual wants to change a behavior to improve health and the intent is high, other non-motivational factors could prevent successful behavior change. The theory of planned behavior as an extension of the theory of reasoned action, addresses this problem. The theory of planned behavior includes the constructs of (1) attitude toward behavior, (2) subjective norm, and (3) perceived behavioral control. The perceived behavioral control reflects the person's belief about the ease or difficulty in performing a behavior, past experiences, and anticipated barriers and obstacles. Perceived behavioral control has motivational implications for behavioral intentions. Perceived behavioral control must be strong for behavioral change to occur. If the attitude toward the behavior and the subjective norm are high and the person's perception of control over the behavior is low, then there is likely to be little success in adopting the new behavior. In matters such as smoking cessation or weight reduction, volition and motivation are not enough. The person must believe that he or she has control over whether or not he or she can really change behaviors for successful health outcomes.

Theory at the Interpersonal Level

Social Cognitive Theory

Social Learning Theory (SLT), as the theory was originally named, explains human behavior in terms of a continuous interaction among cognitive, behavioral and environmental determinants (Parcel and Baranowski, 1981). SLT proposed that a person's behaviors are responses to which other people apply reinforcements. Reinforcement can be used to change a person's behavior directly or vicariously by observing others being rewarded for their behavior and then copying their rewarded behavior. Bandura and Walters (1963) concluded that individuals change their behaviors because they desire to emulate role models who are being rewarded for their behaviors. While there are several versions of the Social Learning Theory, there are basic tenets.

1. Response consequences (such as rewards or punishments) influence the likelihood that a person will repeat a particular behavior in a given situation.

2. Humans can learn by observing others, and they also learn by participating in an act personally. Learning by observing others is called vicarious learning.

3. Individuals are most likely to model behavior that they observe in others with whom they identify and respect. Identification with others is a function of the degree to which a person is perceived to be similar to one's self, in addition to the degree of emotional attachment that is felt toward an individual.

Albert Bandura added to the theory, the constructs of self-efficacy, modeling or vicarious learning, reciprocal determinism, and that there can be significant temporal variation in time lapse between cause and effect. Through Bandura's work (1986), his version of Social Learning Theory became known as Social Cognitive Theory (SCT). Bandura (1986) stated that the Social Cognitive Theory expresses learning to be an internal mental process (cognitive process) that may or may not be reflected in immediate behavioral change. SCT considers the role of personal factors (e.g., beliefs, attitudes, expectations, and memory) in addition to the environmental and behavioral aspects of learning. SCT approaches human behavior in terms of a continuous interaction among personal, behavioral, and environmental determinants. An underlying assumption is that behavior is dynamic and depends on the environment and personal constructs which influence each other simultaneously. The continuing interaction among a person, his or her behavior, and the environment is called *reciprocal determinism* and is illustrated in Figure 6.4.

Figure 6.4 Reciprocal Determinism: Interactional, triadic, reciprocal model between environment, personal factors, and behavior

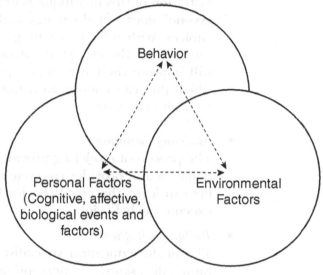

Bandura introduced constructs for application in SCT. These are especially important in health promotion interventions. See Table 6.2.

Table 6.2 Social Cognitive Constructs and Definitions.

SCT constructs	Definitions
Knowledge	The learning of facts and gaining greater insights related to an action, idea, object, person, or situation
Outcome expectations	The anticipation of the desired outcomes that would follow as a result of engaging in the behavior that is being addressed
Outcome expectancies	The value that a person places on the probable outcomes
Situational perception	How one perceives and interprets the environment or situation in which one is surrounded
Environment	The physical and social circumstances in the environment that surrounds a person
Self-efficacy	The confidence in one's ability to establish or change a behavior
Self-efficacy in overcoming impediments	The confidence that one has in overcoming barriers while performing the targeted behavior
Goal setting or self-control	The ability to set goals for chosen behaviors and developing plans to accomplish these goals
Emotional coping	The techniques that one uses to control emotional and physiological challenges associated with the establishment of new behaviors

A number of techniques based on SCT have been developed and have been determined to be effective in health education and health promotion for inducing behavior change (Butler, 2001).

- *Revising expectations*
  This technique involves helping individuals and populations revise how they view outcomes of their behaviors realistically. An illustration of this technique is in helping adolescents see that "everyone" does not do drugs and that they can make different choices. With reliable learning experiences and new knowledge, they will see the expected outcomes of refraining from drug use will improve their health and provide greater life options from which they can choose. Revising expectations is commonly used by health educators.

- *Modeling (imitation)*
  The process of modeling provides knowledge about the healthful behavior and provides concrete examples of how to do it. Learners can learn the new behavior by observing others successfully execute the behavior.

- *Building self-efficacy*
  The health education specialist must be aware of the learner's knowledge, skills, and perceptions of their abilities. Using this information, the learner is assisted in setting realistic goals for developing new behaviors. The learner's process for behavior change is taking small steps to accomplish the goal. Each step enables the learner to be successful and grow in self-efficacy.

- *Contracting*
  In this technique, the learner and at least one other person agree by written contract to achieve a specific behavior. Specific conditions for successful completion of the contract are indicated: the specific behaviors, conditions for measuring successful completion and fulfillment of contract terms, the timeframe, rewards or consequences. This technique usually requires recordkeeping by the participants and the health education specialist.

- *Self-monitoring*
  Self-monitoring is one technique that requires the learner to think about the processes required to achieve behavior change and to set realistic goals. The learner must then monitor his or her progress in achieving the targeted behavior. Self-monitoring is actually like having a contract with oneself.

Theory at the Community Level

Health education/promotion professionals will plan what they believe is an effective program and will want to be sure that the target population will participate in the program for its duration. Therefore health education specialists require skills in marketing and psychology in order to attract the target population and keep them involved in order for behavior change to occur. In marketing a product, the process would come down to offering benefits that the consumer is willing to pay a price for and with which the consumer would be satisfied. In health promotion, program planners would like to exchange costs and benefits with those in the target population. Health educators would like to exchange the benefits of participation in health promotion programs (the objectives or outcomes of the programs they planned) for the costs of the program, which come from the participants, such as their time, money, and effort. Unlike applying marketing principles to a line of clothing or a new car, health promotion programs are health enhancement programs that do not have material objects, but instead they market awareness, knowledge, attitudes, skills, and behavior. For this reason, the marketing of health promotion programs falls into a special type of marketing called social marketing.

Social Marketing

Social marketing, while based on commercial marketing principles, is indeed different when applied to health education and health promotion. Social marketing is a process for influencing human behavior for the purpose of benefiting society and not for commercial purposes or profit. It is used in a variety of situations to influence behaviors and choices on a large scale. In health promotion it can be used to influence the use of health education programs, increase health care utilization, or to communicate campaigns to encourage individuals and groups to change attitudes and behaviors.

Social marketing process is used for planning programs or interventions for large defined populations and its process is similar to the traditional health education program planning process. While there are some differences in terminology, both processes include assessment of potential consumers or target audience, setting specific goals and objectives, planning, implementing, evaluating, and modifying the intervention or campaign. The marketing concepts used in social marketing are consumer orientation, exchange or exchange theory, market segmentation and consumer analysis, demand, competition, the marketing mix, positioning, consumer satisfaction, and brand loyalty (Bensley and Brookins-Fisher, 2009).

Consumer orientation means that the health education specialist or planner is focused on meeting the needs and desires of the consumers in the process of helping them achieve behavior change. In health education, the most important activity is learning as much as possible about the consumer. The health educator must remember that consumers make voluntary choices about changing behaviors or making choices among competing products, offerings and ideas. The more that is known and honored about the consumers will influence the voluntary choices that they make and the success of the programs or services.

Exchange theory implies the transfer or transaction of something valuable between two individuals or groups. In social marketing, the emphasis of this transaction is voluntary and underscores the benefits to the consumer. If a program's participants are encouraged to increase physical activity, the costs to the participants might be their loss of family time, loss of time for television watching, loss of free time, and money paid for transportation to the program site, etc. The benefits for their increased physical activity must be more attractive than the costs. These benefits may be feeling healthier, having more energy, desired weight loss, etc.

Market segmentation or audience segmentation and consumer analysis is central to a social marketing plan. The social marketer identifies distinct groups of people or segments who are similar to each other in various characteristics and are expected to respond to messages in similar ways. These segments may be based on geographic factors, demographic factors, medical history factors, personality characteristics, attitudinal factors, behavioral factors, etc. After identifying the segments, knowledge, attitude, and behavior data are collected from the target audience by using qualitative methods such as focus groups, in-depth interviews, case studies, or quantitative studies using surveys.

The key constructs in social marketing are product, price, place, and promotion and are also referred to as the marketing mix. Product is the desired behavior or offering that is intended for the target audience or consumers to adopt. Price is the tangible and/or the intangible things that the consumer has to give up in order to adopt the new idea or product. Place is where the target audience will perform the behavior. Promotion is the mechanism or methods by which the health education specialist gets the message across to the consumers. A promotion may include a mix of advertising in various media formats, incentives, face to face selling by spokespersons, and public relations that are best suited for the consumers.

Experts in the field of social marketing have added other constructs to the marketing mix that address the social and non-profit funding base of social marketing. These components include publics, partnership, policy, and purse strings.

Publics refer to the primary and secondary external and internal stakeholders that must be considered in planning a social marketing campaign that seeks to change behavior. Partnership addresses the importance of collaborating and partnering with other organizations that can bring expertise and resources to complex problems. Policy relates to the laws, and policies that can affect the context and environment in which the behavioral change must occur. Purse strings deal with various funding sources that are needed to support the social marketing campaign.

Other constructs to be considered in the social marketing campaign are positioning, consumer satisfaction and brand loyalty. In commercial marketing, positioning is creating a personality for the product that the consumer recognizes and expects to take care of their need or problem effectively. The same is true for positioning in social marketing. The proper positioning becomes clear to the planners as they learn about the consumers and their needs, desires, and resources. Consumer satisfaction is the goal of social marketing. Consumers want at least what they expect from the product or service and more than they expect is even better. Satisfied consumers will share their positive experiences with others. Dissatisfied consumers will also share their negative experiences with others. Brand loyalty is the consistent selection and preference for a particular product or service that has proven itself to be effective, satisfactory and reliable over time.

Andreasen (1995) reminds those who design social marketing campaigns that the process is challenging. He recommends six stages for social marketing for producing successful campaigns:

1. *Listening stage* in which background analysis and listening to the target audience is done (the assessment stage).
2. *Planning stage* in which the marketing mission, goals, objectives, and strategy are clearly defined.
3. *Structuring stage* in which marketing organization, procedures, benchmarks, and feedback mechanisms are established.
4. *Pretesting stage* in which key program elements are tested.
5. *Implementing stage* in which the strategy is put into effect.
6. *Monitoring stage* in which program progress is tracked and evaluated.

These stages for social marketing are very similar to the health education process that will be presented later in this textbook.

Diffusion of Innovations Theory

Diffusion of Innovation theory is strongly based in marketing theory, but also involves the communication channels necessary to promote an innovation. Diffusion refers to the process by which new ideas, objects or practice are adopted by individuals in target populations. Diffusion theories view communication as a two-way process, rather than one of merely "persuading" an audience to take action. There is a two-step flow of communication, in which opinion leaders mediate the impact of mass media and emphasize the value of social networks, or interpersonal channels, over and above mass media, for adoption decisions. For an example, health professionals and community leaders are especially important allies and communication channels for new ideas, practices, programs and products to improve health. As they repeat the same information that is provided through mass media channels, the chances that the target audience will act positively toward the innovation increases.

There are four constructs in the diffusion of innovations theory (Rogers, 2003). The first is innovation. Innovations are new ideas, practices, services, or products that are offered to individuals and groups who perceive them as new. It does not matter how long the idea, product or practice has existed, what is important is that the target population views it as new. A limited number of attributes for an innovation are presented in Table 6.3.

Table 6.3 Attributes of Innovations

Attributes	Definition	Application
Relative Advantage	The degree to which an innovation is seen as better than the idea, practice, program, or product it replaces	Point out unique benefits: monetary value convenience, time saving, prestige, etc.
Compatibility	How consistent the innovation is with values, habits, experience, and needs of potential adopters	Tailor innovation for the intended audience's values, norms, or situation.
Complexity	How difficult the innovation is to understand and/or use	Create program/idea/product to be uncomplicated, easy to use and understand.
Trialability	Extent to which the innovation can be experimented with before a commitment to adopt is required	Provide opportunities to try on a limited basis, e.g., free samples, introductory sessions, money-back guarantee.
Observability	Extent to which the innovation provides tangible or visible results	Assure visibility of results: feedback or publicity.

The second construct is communication channels. Communication channels are the links between those who have knowledge and expertise regarding the innovation and the individuals and population who have not adopted the innovation. Time is the third construct. Time is the interval between the target population's awareness of the innovation and the adoption of the innovation. Finally, the fourth construct for this theory is social system, which addresses how people relate to each other as individuals, families, groups, organizations, and communities. In this theory it is important to know how similar group members are. Similarity of group members is homophily. Innovations generally spread faster among individuals and groups that have much in common and are more similar, enhancing the diffusion of the innovation.

Other aspects of the social system are the social networks, change agent, and opinion leaders. Social networks are physical or virtual person-centered webs of social relationships that lend support, friendship and communication. Social networks may actually govern the pace at which innovations are adopted. The change agent is the person who positively influences the potential adopter. This person or persons may be the health education specialist or other influential health provider. Change agents will be involved in promoting the intervention and innovation. Opinion leaders are individuals who are influential in communities and can effectively influence the beliefs and actions of their colleagues, positively or negatively. Opinion leaders' support should be solicited early and they should be recruited to the program early.

Diffusion theory can demonstrate the process of marketing innovations or health promotion interventions, as health education specialists examine how their program will be adopted. When the consumers adopt an innovation they are referred to as adopters.

Rogers (1983) explained the diffusion of innovation in populations, or the adoption patterns of the innovation by adopters, based on when

Figure 6.5 Adopter categories and the bell-shaped curve

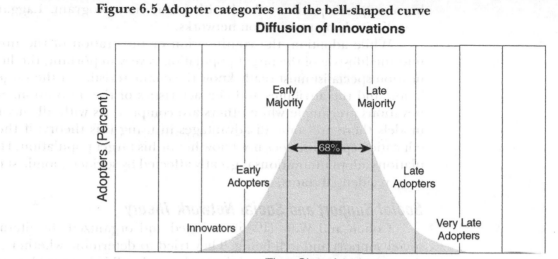

they adopt innovations. Rogers used a bell-shaped curve divided into adopter categories to describe this phenomenon.

The value of the diffusion theory in health promotion programs is its ability to distinguish the characteristics of people in the target population and consistently predict how people will participate in the health promotion innovations. The diffusion of innovation theory, as represented by the normal bell-shaped curve, identifies innovators as those persons who fall in the portion of the curve that is left of -2 standard deviations from the mean. Innovators who are 2% to 3% of the target population would probably become involved with a health program because they heard about it and wanted to be the first participants. They are usually ahead of their time.

Early adopters represent about 14% of the target population, -2 to -1 standard deviations on the curve. Early adopters are those people who are usually interested in the innovation, but they are not the first to sign up. They usually wait on the innovators so that they can be sure the innovation is useful. Early adopters are seen as opinion leaders by the target population and respected by that population.

The next two groups, early majority and late majority, represent between -1 standard deviation and the mean and between the mean and +1 standard deviation. Each of these groups is about 34% of the target population. The early majority takes more time to deliberate before making a decision. The late majority takes even more time for making the decision, because they are more skeptical and are not likely to become involved until most members of the target population are participating in the health promotion program.

The late adopters and the very late adopters, also known as laggards, are the 16% of the target population represented by the part of the curve greater than +1 standard deviation. Laggards are not usually interested in new innovations, so they would be the last to participate. The very late adopters are also populations that are hard to reach. They may not even become participants in the health promotion program. Laggards may have limited communication networks.

While adoption, the continuation or integration of the innovation into the lifestyle of the target population is very important, the health education specialist must really know the characteristics of the target population and the attributes and characteristics of the innovation. Some innovations are simple while others are complex. As with all theories and models there are some disadvantages in using this theory, if the health education specialist does not know her or his target population. How populations adopt innovations is greatly affected by socioeconomic status, culture, residential status, etc.

Social Support and Social Network Theory

Cohen and Wills (1985) reviewed and organized the literature on social support and well-being. They tried to determine whether the positive association between social support and well-being may be attributed more to an overall beneficial effect of support (director model) or to a process of support that protects persons from the potentially adverse effects of stressful events (buffering model). The research studies were divided by whether a measure assesses support structure (the existence of relationships) or function (the extent to which one's interpersonal relationships provide particular resources).

Numerous studies have demonstrated that the extent and nature of one's social relationships affect one's health (House et. al., 1988). An understanding of the impact of social relationships on health status, health behaviors, and health decision-making can contribute greatly to the development of effective interventions for preventing the onset of diseases and promoting health. Various conceptual models and theories have guided research in this area, but there is no one theory or model that actually explains the linkage. Social network is a person-centered web of social relationships. The provision of social support is one of the important functions of social relationships. Therefore social networks are linkages between people that may (or may not) provide social support and that may serve other functions in addition to support.

The structure of social networks can be described in terms of characteristics such as:

- **Reciprocity:** the extent to which resources and support are both given and received in a relationship

- **Intensity:** the extent to which a relationship is characterized by emotional closeness

- **Complexity:** the extent to which a relationship serves a variety of functions

- **Homogeneity:** the extent to which network members are similar in terms of demographic characteristics such as age, race, and socioeconomic status

- **Geographical dispersion:** the extent to which network members live in close proximity to the focal person

  - **Density:** the extent to which network members know and interact with each other

House (1981) defined social support by the functional content of relationships.

- **Emotional support:** the provision of empathy, love, trust, and caring

- **Instrumental support:** provides tangible aid and services, that directly assists a person in need

- **Informational support:** provides advice, suggestions, and information that a person can use in problem-solving

- **Appraisal support:** provides information that is useful for self-evaluation purposes that is constructive feedback, affirmation, and social comparison

While the four types of support can be presented conceptually as separate, in reality relationships that offer one type of support will also provide the other types of support. Heaney and Israel (1997) hypothesized a direct interplay of social networks and physical, mental and social health, each affecting the other in a bidirectional feedback loop. They reasoned that social networks would offer persons close relationships and the esteem of others, a sense of belonging, and self-esteem that would tend to improve health regardless of the effects of other factors on health. Similarly, they hypothesized that individual coping resources, organizational and community resources, and health behaviors would also have a bidirectional interplay with health. Furthermore, the degree of individual coping resources would affect stress, and so would the degree of organizational/community resources. Individual coping resources might include the ability to problem-solve, to access new contacts and information, and increased perceived control. Organizational/community resources might be reflected in community empowerment.

Heaney and Israel (1997) proposed that strengthening social networks and enhancing the exchange of social support may increase a community's ability to garner its resources and solve problems. The work by Minkler (1990) and Eng and Parker (1994) documented that several community interventions have shown how intentional network building and strengthening social support within communities are associated with enhanced community capacity and control for changes in health status. The availability of improved individual or community resources increases the likelihood that stressors will be dealt with so that adverse health consequences are reduced. This is known as the buffering effect. Also, social networks and social support may mediate the frequency and duration of exposure to stressors. Finally, social networks and social support have potential effects on health behaviors. By mediating behavioral risk factors, preventive health practices and illness behaviors, social networks, and social support may have an impact on the incidence of, diagnosis of, and recovery from disease.

The use of social support and social network theory can help the health professional in designing effective interventions and methods to change health behaviors and health status for individuals and communities. Heaney and Israel (1997) suggest the following types of possible social network interventions with examples of activities and methods.

- *Enhancing existing social network linkages:* training of network members in skills for support provision; training of indigenous individuals in mobilizing and maintaining social networks; systems approach (i.e., marital counseling, family therapy, mediation services, etc.)

- *Developing new social network linkages:* creating linkages to mentors; developing buddy systems; coordinating self-help groups

- *Enhancing networks through the use of indigenous natural helpers:* identification of natural helpers in the community; analysis of natural helpers' existing social networks; training of natural helpers in health topics and community problem-solving strategies

- *Enhancing networks at the community level through participatory problem-solving:* Identification of overlapping networks within the community; examination of social network characteristics of members of the selected need or target area; facilitation of ongoing community problem identification and problem-solving

Health professionals have effectively used these interventions to identify, recruit and train people who are natural helpers in the target population and assist individuals in a specific social network and community. The natural helpers are often referred to as lay health advisors or community health advisors. They are trained to provide information on specific health issues, information on and access to health and community resources and services, emotional support, and provide leadership in community problem solving.

A Framework for Planning Practice and Research

Frameworks are planning tools, which incorporate theories or models or parts of them. One of the most popular of the planning frameworks used in health education/promotion program planning is the PRECEDE-PROCEED Model. While there are other frameworks and models that can be used for program planning, PRECEDE-PROCEED is one of the well-developed planning tools that can be used to integrate diverse theoretical frameworks.

PRECEDE-PROCEED Model

Green and Kreuter (2005) designed PRECEDE-PROCEED as a planning model for health education and health promotion programs. It is an ecological approach to planning for health promotion interventions. The model originated in the 1970s. The acronym PRECEDE stands for predisposing, reinforcing, and enabling causes in educational diagnosis and evaluation. PROCEED is the acronym for policy, regulatory, and organizational constructs in education and environmental development. One of the strong principles upon which the model is based is the principle of participation. The principle emphasizes active participation of the target audience in defining their own issues, priorities, and goals in developing and implementing solutions for those issues. Achieving healthy behavioral change is greatly enhanced by the active participation of the target population. At every phase of the model, the health professional must include the target population (Green and Kreuter, 1991). In 2005, PRECEDE-PROCEED model was updated and now has eight phases in the planning process instead of the nine original phases in the planning process (Green and Kreuter, 2005). According to Green and Kreuter (2005, p. 18), the most important hallmarks of the PRECEDE-PROCEED Model are: "(1) flexibility and scalability, (2) evidence–based process and evaluability, (3) its commitment to the principle of participation, and (4) its provision of a process for appropriate adaptation of evidence-based 'best practices'. "

Figure 6.6 PRECEDE-PROCEED Model

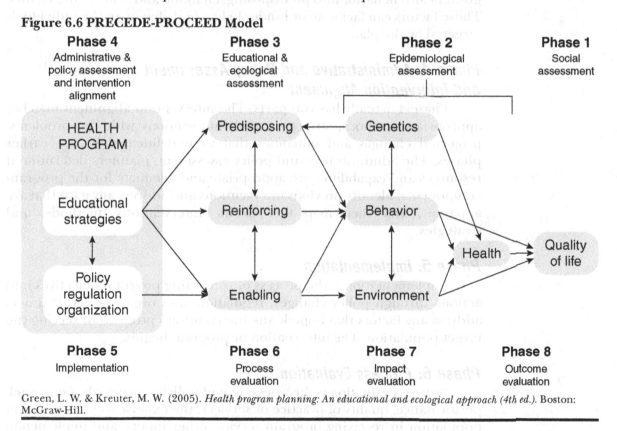

Green, L. W. & Kreuter, M. W. (2005). *Health program planning: An educational and ecological approach (4th ed.).* Boston: McGraw-Hill.

Phase 1: Social Assessment

The social assessment phase assesses the quality of life in a community. The social assessment looks at both the objective and subjective data that reveals high-priority problems and/or aspirations for the common good of the population. From both primary and secondary data, economic and social indicators and the population's documentation define the individuals' and community's quality of life.

Phase 2: Epidemiological Assessment

The epidemiological assessment phase delineates the extent, distribution, and causes of a health problem found in the defined population. The planners use data to identify and rank health goals or problems that may contribute to problems identified in phase 1. This phase includes mortality, morbidity, and disability data as well as genetic, behavioral, and environmental factors. It is important that planners rank the health problems because there are rarely enough resources to address all problems.

Phase 3: Educational and Ecological Assessment

The educational and ecological assessment is the explanation of the specific health-related actions that will most likely cause positive health outcomes. Phase 3 identifies and classifies factors that can influence a given health behavior into predisposing, enabling and reinforcing factors. These factors can facilitate or hinder behavioral change in the individuals targeted by the plan.

Phase 4: Administrative and Policy Assessment and Intervention Alignment

Phase 4 actually has two parts. The intervention alignment matches appropriate methods, strategies, and interventions with the problems, projected changes and outcomes that were delineated in the earlier phases. The administrative and policy assessment, planners determine if resources and capabilities are appropriate and adequate for the program components, identify previous interventions and address any gaps that are apparent, and then map the specific interventions, methods, and strategies.

Phase 5: Implementation

Implementation is the process of converting program objectives into actions through policy changes, regulation, and organization. Planners address any factors that impede the intervention's progress in serving the target population. The intervention or program begins.

Phase 6: Process Evaluation

Process evaluation is the assessment of policies, materials, personnel, performance, quality of practice or services, the experiences of the target population in receiving program service, other inputs, and implementation experiences.

Phase 7: Impact Evaluation

Impact evaluation assesses immediate effects of the intervention on targeted behaviors and/or environments. The impact assessment determines program effects on intermediate objectives that include changes in predisposing, enabling, and reinforcing factors.

Phase 8: Outcome Evaluation

Outcome evaluation determines the effects of the program on its ultimate objectives, including changes in health, social benefits and/or the quality of life.

The health education specialists have major responsibilities for planning, implementing and evaluating health education and health promotion interventions. Planning models certainly help the professionals effectively and efficiently fulfill these responsibilities. Planning models like the PRECEDE-PROCEED Model help the planner to grasp three fundamental assumptions: (1) all planning must begin with appropriate assessments; (2) health and health risks have multiple causes and (3) efforts to address health and health risk change must be multilevel and multidimensional.

References

Andreasen, A. R. 1994. "Social Marketing: Its Definition and Domain." *Journal of Public Policy & Marketing* 13 (1): 108–114.

Bandura, A., and R. H. Walters. 1963. *Social Learning and Personality Development*. New York: Holt, Rinehart and Winston.

Bandura, A. 2004. "Health Promotion by Social Cognitive Means." *Health Education and Behavior* 31: 143–64.

Bensley, R. J. and J. Brookins-Fisher (editors). 2009. *Community Health Education Methods: A Practical Guide (3rd edition)*. Sudbury: Jones and Bartlett Publishers.

Butler, J. T. 1997. *Principles of Health Education and Health Promotion (2nd edition)*. Englewood: Morton Publishing Company.

Butler, J. T. 2001. *Principles of Health Education and Health Promotion, 3rd ed*. Belmont, CA: Wadsworth/Thomas Learning.

Cohen, S., and T. A. Wills. 1985. "Stress, Social Support, and the Buffering Hypothesis." *Psychological Bulletin* 98 (2): 310–57.

Coreil, J. 2010. Social and Behavioral Foundations of Public Health. Los Angeles: Sage Publications, Inc.

Cottrell, R. R., J. T. Girvan, and J. F. McKenzie. 2012. *Principles and Foundations of Health Promotion and Education*. Boston: Benjamin Cummings.

Eng, E., and E. Parker. 1994. "Measuring Community Competence in the Mississippi Delta: The Interface Between Program Evaluation and Empowerment." *Health Education and Behavior* 21 (2): 199–220.

Fishbein, M. and I. Ajzen. 1975. *Beliefs, Attitudes, Intention and Behavior: An Introduction to Theory and Research*. Reading MA: Addison-Wesley.

Gilbert, G. G., R. G. Sawyer, & E. B. McNeill. 2011. *Health Education: Creating Strategies for School and Community Health (3rd edition)*. Sudbury: Jones and Bartlett Publishers.

Glanz, K., F. M. Lewis, & B. K. Rimer (Eds.). 1997. *Health Behavior and Health Education: Theory, research, and practice (2nd edition)*. San Francisco: Jossey-Bass.

Glanz, K., and B. K. Rimer. 2005. *Theory at a Glance: A Guide for Health Promotion Practice*. National Cancer Institute, National Institutes of Health, US Department of Health and Human Services. NIH Pub. No. 97–3896. Washington, DC: NIH.

Green, L. W., and M. W. Kreuter. 1999. *Health Promotion Planning: An Educational and Ecological Approach*, 3rd ed. San Francisco, CA : Mayfield.

Green, L. W., and M. W. Kreuter. 2005. *Health Program Planning: An Educational and Ecological Approach*, 4th ed. Boston: McGraw-Hill.

Hanson, D., J. Hanson, P. Vardon, K. MacFarlane, J. Lloyd, R. Muller, et al. 2005. "The Injury Iceberg: An Ecological Approach to Planning Sustainable Community Safety Interventions." *Health Promotion Journal of Australia* 16 (1): 5–10.

Heaney, C. A., and B. A. Israel. 1997. Social Support and Social Networks. In K. Glanz, B. Rimer, and F. Lewis, eds. *Health Behavior and Health Education: Theory, Research, and Practice*, 2nd ed. San Francisco, CA: Jossey-Bass, pp. 179–205.

House, J. S., D. Umberson, and K. R. Landis. 1988. "Social Relationships and Health." *Science* 241 (4865): 540–45.

House, J. S., D. Umberson, and K. R. Landis. 1988. Structures and Processes of Social Support. *Annual Review of Sociology* 14: 293–318.

Janz, N. K., and M. H. Becker. 1984. "The Health Belief Model—A Decade Later." *Health Education Quarterly* 11 (1): 1–47.

Ledlow, G. R., and M. N. Coppola. 2011. Leadership for Health Professionals: Theory, Skills, and Applications. Sudbury, MA: Jones & Barlett Learning.

McKenzie, J. F., and J. L. Smeltzer. 1997. *Planning, Implementing, and Evaluating Health Promotion Programs: A Primer (2nd edition)*. Boston: Allyn and Bacon.

McKenzie, J. F., and J. L. Smeltzer. 2001. *Planning, Implementing, and Evaluating Health Promotion Programs: A Primer*, 3rd ed. New York: Macmillan.

McKenzie, J. F., B. L. Neiger, and R. Thackeray. 2013. *Planning, Implementing, and Evaluating Health Education Programs: A Primer*. Boston: Pearson Education.

Minkler, M. 1990. "Improving Health Through Community Organization." In K. Glanz, F. M. Lewis, and B. Rimer, eds. *Health Behavior and Health Education: Theory, Research, and Practice*. (pp. 257–287). San Francisco, CA: Jossey-Bass.

Parcel and Baranowski. 1981. "Social Learning Theory and Health Education." *Health Education* 12 (3): 14–18.

Prochaska, J. O. 1979. *Systems of Psychotherapy: A Transtheoretical analysis*. Homewood, IL: Dorsey Press.

Prochaska, J. O., & DiClemente, C. C. 1983. "Stages and Processes of Self-change of Smoking: Toward an integrative model of change." *Journal of Consulting and Clinical Psychology* 51 (3): 390–395.

Prochaska, J. O., DiClemente, C. C., & Norcross, J. C. 1992. "In Search of How People Change: Applications to Addictive Behaviors." *American Psychologist* 47 (9): 1102–1114.

Prochaska, J. O., & W. F. Velicer. 1997. "Introduction: The Transtheoretical Model." *American Journal of Health Promotion* 12 (1): 6–7.

Rogers, E. M. 1983. *Diffusion of Innovations*, 3rd ed. New York: Free Press.

Rogers, E. M. 2003. *Diffusion of Innovations*, 5th ed. New York: Free Press.

Rosenstock, I. M., V. J. Strecher, and M. H. Becker. 1988. "Why People use Health Services." *Milbank Memorial Fund Quarterly* 15 (2): 175–183.

Sharma, M., and J. A. Romas. 2012. Theoretical Foundations of Health Education and Health Promotion, 2nd. ed. Sudbury, MA: Jones & Barlett Learning.

Wills, T. A. 1985. Supportive Functions of Interpersonal Relationships. In S. Cohen & L. Syme. Social support and health. pp. 61–82. Orlando, FL: Academic Press.

Chapter 7

The Health Education Process for Healthy Behavior Change and Needs Assessment

Figure 7.1 Health Education Process for Improved Quality of Life

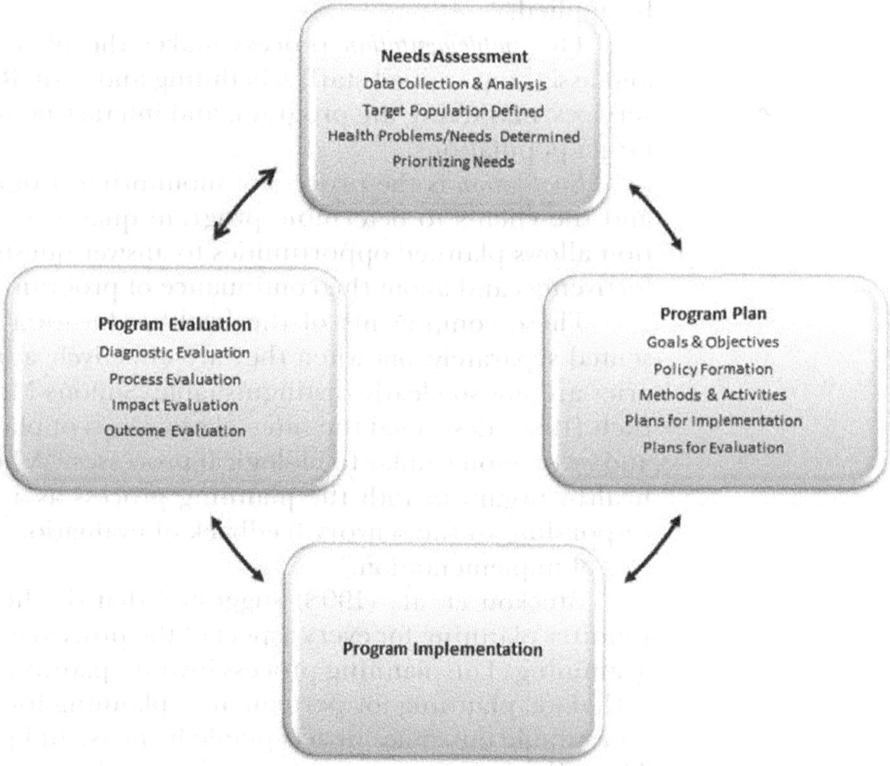

Needs Assessment
Data Collection & Analysis
Target Population Defined
Health Problems/Needs Determined
Prioritizing Needs

Program Evaluation
Diagnostic Evaluation
Process Evaluation
Impact Evaluation
Outcome Evaluation

Program Plan
Goals & Objectives
Policy Formation
Methods & Activities
Plans for Implementation
Plans for Evaluation

Program Implementation

The health education process is at the core of behavior changes for successful health impacts and outcomes that improve health and the quality of life. The health education process includes needs assessment, program planning, program implementation, and program evaluation. The health education specialist has great responsibility in producing effective programs and interventions that result in responsible behavior change for improved health and quality of life. In fact, these components of the process represent four of the areas of responsibility for the health education specialists. Successful program development and intervention is dependent upon effective needs assessment, planning, implementation, and evaluation.

Needs assessment is the process by which the health education specialist identifies the issues, the needs, and problems that challenge our citizens and communities. The needs assessment identifies the target population most affected by the problems and their characteristics. The needs assessment also includes the identification of resources that individuals and populations can bring to meet their challenges.

Program planning is the process of determining the most effective ways to address the problems and needs of the target population who are most affected by the problems and who will receive the services to be offered; the nature of the services to be offered; and how resources should be applied.

The *implementation* process makes the plan reality through hiring and assigning trained staff; scheduling and actually offering the program services; marketing the program, and interacting with the consumers and target populations.

Evaluation is the process of monitoring program resources, services and the clients to determine program quality and effectiveness. Evaluation allows planned opportunities to answer questions about program effectiveness and about the continuance of program activities.

These components of the health education process are often presented separately, but when they are effectively administered, the boundaries are not so clearly distinguishable. Simons-Morton, Greene and Gottlieb (1995) described the interrelationships of planning, implementation and evaluation similar to biological processes: "A healthy program is like a healthy organism with the planning process as a central nervous system responding to the sensory feedback of evaluation and directing the muscles of implementation."

Breckon et. al., (1998) suggested that the health education process requires planning for every aspect of the process for health education programming. The planning process involves planning with people, planning with data, planning for permanence, planning for priorities, planning for measurable outcomes in acceptable formats, and planning for evaluation. The following gives an overview of these planning concerns which are included in the process.

Plan with people. The people involved with the planning team must include representatives from the target population who are respected by the community, opinion leaders, and competent and trusted health professionals.

Plan the needs assessment process. The planners must determine the kinds of information and data that will be necessary to do effective program planning and how it will be collected, and by whom it will be collected and reported.

Plan with data. The data gathered through the needs assessment will be critical in directing the planning process. It is central to identifying health problems, issues, and resources.

Plan the program implementation. Planning is required in the effective selection and training of program staff, the marketing of the program, the recruitment of participants, the quality of services to the target population, the building of collaborations and partnerships, and in the administration of the program.

Plan the program evaluation. An effective plan for the program will provide for systematic and timely collection and analysis of information for successful program performance and decision-making.

Plan for dissemination of program progress, results and reports. Several individuals and groups must be involved and informed in the progress and outcomes of the program, such as the planners, their supervisors, administrators, community leaders, funding organizations, the target population, cooperating community agencies and organizations, etc.

Needs Assessment

The first important task of program planning is the *needs assessment.* The needs assessment allows for the examination of the health status of persons, specific groups, or the community, the identification of problems or issues, and the related factors. Perhaps the best definition for needs assessment is the process by which the health professional determines and measures the gaps between the population's health needs and the health care and health promotion services available to improve the population's health. Needs assessment is actually part of the evaluation and is also known as the diagnostic evaluation in program evaluation. This part of the planning process involves the collection of data that helps to identify individual, family and community resources, assets, and community stakeholders and leadership. The health education specialist and the planning committee must determine the purpose and scope of the needs assessment. What is to be gained by the assessment? Assessments can be informal and simple or formal and complex. This decision usually will be based on resources available and the expertise of the professional staff.

The needs assessment is that part of the planning process that serves to identify a population's most critical health issues and problems. The needs assessment is a planned effort to become acquainted with the population, their community setting, and the environment. The assessment presents the health education specialist with the opportunity to know the population's needs and issues, existing resources, the gaps between the needs and the resources, before recommending solutions and actions. The needs assessment includes both formal and informal data collection. It also includes the perceptions and values of the community leaders, groups, agencies, individuals and health organizations' staff about the health issues, problems, assets, barriers, and priorities for a given population. The data that is collected can include specific data and survey information to identify and verify the health status of a given population and the level of risk for that population. Without the needs assessment, there is no way to determine what services, programs, and policies are needed for which populations. While the needs assessment is used as the logical starting point of program planning, it is also an important method for monitoring change within the population being studied.

Who is Involved in the Needs Assessment?

The practitioners of health education and health promotion focus on the goal of helping people (individuals, families, groups, and communities) choose patterns of behaviors which move them toward optimal health rather than toward disease. The goal includes helping these people to have the abilities to avoid many of the imbalances, diseases, and accidents of life. Therefore it is very important that the people who will receive the intervention and those who will be involved in the planning and implementation of the intervention work together in the overall planning process. The individuals who will be involved in the program must be involved *actively* in the planning—from conception through evaluation. The following individuals and groups should be considered as active participants in the process:

- Community members who will be clients/consumers
- Community leaders and stakeholders
- Health professionals serving the specific community
- Community elders
- Spiritual leaders
- Professionals officially responsible for the program plan

The health education specialist may actually select and recruit members of the above community groups and establish an advisory group for the project.

Health education specialists find community involvement very helpful and important in the health education process. Unfortunately, in many programs and services, there has been little, if any, community or tribal participation beyond the data collection. The results of not including representatives of the target population and the community throughout the process are that problems are poorly defined; the intervention misses the community context of the issues; the cultural context for the intervention is often missing; and the findings, conclusions, and assumptions are often incomplete, if not erroneous. Community involvement in the intervention usually means that problems such as trust issues and the lack of understanding among the target group to receive services, can be avoided. This growing role for community participation can also lead to the growing emphasis on self-determination in many communities, community empowerment, and the elimination of controversial and stigmatizing research and intervention outcomes that may produce negative stereotypes. Community members can help health education and health promotion professionals identify the differences between the values of the dominant culture and those of other cultures that can dictate the success for programs.

The relationships that planners and researchers have with the individuals, groups, and communities with whom they work must be firmly grounded in mutual respect, trust, and honesty. The quality of these relationships requires health education specialists to work with various populations from varied races, ethnicities, values, belief systems, spiritual and religious backgrounds, and genders. It is vital that health education specialists are culturally sensitive and culturally competent in the execution of all responsibilities and services. Cultural competence is central to developing trusting and respectful relationships. The health education specialist is expected to provide learning opportunities and experiences to help the population receiving services to also develop cultural competence so that they can better navigate the health care systems to receive appropriate and needed services. The Joint Committee on Terminology in Health Education and Health Promotion (2012, p. 16) defines cultural competence as "A developmental process defined as a set of values, principles, behaviors, attitudes, and policies that enable health professionals to work effectively across racial, ethnic and linguistically diverse populations."

Target Population

All of the information collected for each of the tasks listed below will contribute to identifying the target population and the issues that the planners will address. The target population is the group that is determined to be at risk for health problems or challenges based on the collected data. The target population is the population group that is being considered and will receive the benefits of the program being planned. It is the health of the target group that becomes the focus of the planned intervention.

Required Tasks for the Needs Assessment

The health professional must have a plan for the needs assessment that includes data collection from a variety of credible sources in order to accomplish the following:

1. Determination of the current health status of the target population.

2. Inventory of community assets and resources available to the community's populations.

3. Determination of the populations' use of existing health services.

4. Perceptions of the health providers regarding the elderly, disabled, maternal, child and youth health needs, since these are usually the most vulnerable population groups. However, other vulnerable and at-risk populations may be identified by the health providers.

5. Perceptions of the community regarding the elderly, disabled, maternal, child and youth health needs, since these are usually the most vulnerable population groups. However, other vulnerable and at-risk populations may be identified by the community.

6. Identification of the variables, factors and indicators from the health system, providers, individuals, families, community and environment that affect the population's health status and the health system.

7. Analysis of the collected data to define the health problem(s) or issue(s).

8. Establishment of priorities for addressing the health problem or issues of the defined target population.

Data Collection: Using the Professional Literature in the Health Education Process

The needs assessment reveals the current conditions, quality of life, and health status of the target population through data collection and analyses. The data collected must reflect the viewpoint of the health professionals and the viewpoint of the target population (perceived or actual needs). The sources of data for a needs assessment are varied and dependent upon the concerns of a given community and the planners.

The health education process requires much knowledge and experience from those responsible for program planning. The target populations and the communities will supply a great amount of credible data that will be important to the planning efforts. However, one of the most important resources that professionals in health education and health promotion can readily access is the vast stores of literature available in print and electronic formats. Not only does this resource help the professional health educator in the planning process, but it also provides the health education specialist with an ever expanding source of information.

This information is important to fulfilling the responsibilities of serving as a health education resource person and advocating for health and health education. There has been an explosion in the health literature that is available, because of the increasing demand to know more about health issues. Needless to say, all health education specialists would be wise to consult with and gain the assistance of a reference librarian (Cottrell et. al., 2012). Fulfilling the areas of responsibility in health education requires accessing and using data. The sources of data used by the health education specialist for the needs assessment may be primary, secondary, or tertiary.

The primary sources of data are eyewitness accounts and studies with data collected personally by the planner that answers unique questions related to specific data needs. Primary data that one personally collects may be from conducted experiments, interviews, focus groups, surveys, questionnaires, or personal records that relate to the topic in question (McKenzie et. al., 2013). Primary data has the advantage of directly addressing questions that health program planners want answered by the target population. However, primary data can be expensive given the time and financial resources that may be required in collecting, analyzing, and reporting the data. Primary research data or information is often published in peer reviewed or referred journals. Many of these journals are available in print or electronic formats. Peer reviewed journals are those which publish articles only after the manuscripts have been reviewed and accepted by panels of experts.

Secondary data are those data already collected and published by someone else and are available for your use. The advantage of using secondary data is that they already exist, so there is minimal time spent in data collection; and accessing secondary data is usually inexpensive. Secondary sources of data are usually published in journals or books. Journals may be peer-reviewed or refereed. Secondary data can also be found in governmental publications and in credible nongovernmental agencies and organizations. These agencies will usually provide formal publications of their data for use by professionals through free print or electronic access. Most colleges and universities serve as repositories for these data sources. Some sources for secondary data include:

- National, state, and local health status and vital statistics annual reports
- Epidemiological data
- County and city information from different organizations, hospitals, and health units
- Records of health and health care
- Health Risk Appraisals or Health Hazard Appraisals
- Historical accounts
- Peer-reviewed research findings and current literature
- Internet sources that are credible (May include websites of professional health organizations that are governmental or nongovernmental)

Tertiary sources of data are data collected from primary and secondary sources and refined to be included in handbooks, manuals, informational brochures serving the purposes of specific agencies or organization. This data would also include that which appears in encyclopedias, almanacs, dictionaries, fact books and other reference sources. Information from these sources is usually regarded as fact by the scientific community (Cottrell et. al., 2012). Information that has no documentation to support its credibility and is replete with opinions intended for marketing a product is not tertiary data. These sources are classified as a fourth type of literature: popular press publications. These are usually magazine articles or editorials which are often biased. Information from the popular press must be scrutinized before confirming them as authentic, accurate or credible.

Because there is such a great need for data in the health education process, it is important that the planner knows how to conduct a literature search. It is fortunate that health education specialists have access to the internet and literature databases. Libraries in universities, colleges, and communities can provide access to databases. Databases can provide comprehensive listings of citations for journal articles, book chapters, books and access to abstracts of the literature. Most databases can identify sources by both author and subject or title. Some of the most common databases used by professionals in health education and health promotion are listed here.

> PubMed or Medline is a database provided by the US National Library of Medicine.
>
> Education Resource Information Center (ERIC) sponsored by the Institute of Education Sciences (IES), US Department of Education.
>
> PsycINFO produced by the American Psychological Association.
>
> Web of Science (Web of Knowledge) sponsored by Thomas Reuters.
>
> EBSCO *host* provided by EBSCO Publishing.
>
> Google Scholar provided by Google.

The following steps should help in a literature search.

Step 1 Identify the data need or topic that is to be searched. Search by subject or title or by author's last name. If the topic cannot be found, use other key words with similar meanings. Use a thesaurus if necessary.

Step 2 Search the topic or author in the database by the publication years of interest.

Step 3 From the results of your search, identify the possible data sources that meet the need or topic.

Step 4 Locate the literature sources in print or electronically.

Step 5 By reviewing the abstracts or the entire document, determine the quality and usefulness of the data sources or publications to the needs assessment process.

Step 6 Examine the references in the article. This may lead the planner to other data sources that may be useful.

Step 7 Keep a listing of all sources with full citations so that it can be easily transferred to the intervention plan's reference list or bibliography. The planner must always cite and reference all data used in the process.

Primary Data Collection Methods

Primary data collection is important because it can provide accurate population-specific data about problems, influences, and potential solutions to health issues. Collecting primary data through surveys, interviews, and focus group interviews can help the health education specialist establish important relationships with the community and its residents. Primary data collection methods are individual assessments and group assessments.

Individual assessments include surveys, the Delphi technique and interviewing. A survey is a structured method of gathering information directly from the individual by asking questions. Answers to questions may be obtained by mailed surveys that are returned by mail. Telephone surveys and face to face surveys are other options. When using survey methods, the health professional must be sure that the data collected is representative of the target population. The planner must address the questions of how the survey sample is chosen, and whether the survey instrument is valid and reliable. The valid survey instrument must measure what it is intended to measure. The reliable survey instrument must provide consistent results with subsequent use.

The Delphi technique is used when objective information is not available from other means. The Delphi technique generates "a consensus of opinion within a group through a series of questions. The process usually involves three to five rounds of mailed questionnaires in which the participants are asked to respond to general questions in the first round. From these responses more specific questions are asked with each successive round. This becomes a good technique to identify goals and establish priorities in a group or to clarify issues important to the group.

The interviewing method is unique and can encourage participation, but it is very dependent on the interviewer's skill in obtaining data from the interviewee. Establishing rapport and trust with the interviewee are key factors.

There are many trade-offs between cost of data collection and quality of the data obtained. The cost of data collection and summarization tends to increase as we move along the spectrum of mail surveys, telephone surveys, face-to-face surveys, interviews, and medical examinations. Butler (2001) notes the advantages and disadvantages of each. To choose a method of data collection, examine the advantages that may include: affordable cost, acceptable time frames, accuracy of data, honesty of answers, privacy and convenience of the respondent, likely rates of return (response or completion rates), degree to which complex vs. standardized questions can be asked, and scientific validity of the resulting data. In-person surveys and interviews may have the added advantages of building trust between the interviewer and interviewee and increasing morale in the community.

On one end of the continuum, mail surveys are relatively quick and inexpensive, and the individual's privacy can be protected, at least on the surveyor's end, so that answers may be more honest. However, the mailing list may be inaccurate, there is no ability to determine who answers the questions, rates of return may be low, and the returned surveys may be incomplete. In addition, questions need to be simple, and there is no opportunity to clarify them for the respondents. On the other end of the continuum, medical examinations are costly, but highly accurate and quantitative. Honoring the privacy of potential respondents and keeping participants' data confidential is very important, and laws about private health information such as the Health Insurance Portability and Accountability Act (HIPAA) may come into play. In every incidence of collecting data, participants must give their informed consent to participate in the data collection protocol.

Whereas standardized surveys and medical examinations may provide quantitative data about groups, key informant interviews allow for in-depth, nuanced, qualitative data which may provide insights into the context and dimensions of issues in the community. Interviewers must be highly trained, and the very richness of the data may make data analysis time-consuming and difficult. This method allows for considerable trust to be built between the interviewer and interviewee, but embarrassing or threatening questions might not be answered accurately.

In between mailed surveys and interviews are telephone and face-to-face surveys. Interviewers can help to assure survey completion, and questions can be somewhat more complex than in mailed surveys. However, key groups may not have telephones, or may not be willing to answer a telephone for this purpose, "interviewer bias" may occur if the interviewer changes the questions, or the subjects may change their answers so as to be more socially acceptable.

The group assessments include nominal group process, focus group interviews and forums. Nominal group process is a highly structured process that allows researchers or planners to qualify and quantify specific needs of a target population. The group consists of five to seven participants who have some understanding of the issues being considered. The members are asked to write their answers to a question without discussion. Each member then shares one response in a round-robin fashion until each response from every member has been heard by the group. Participants then vote to select and rank the number of items they think are most important related to the issue of concern.

Focus group interviews first began as a method in group therapy. It then evolved as a marketing technique that seeks to understand consumer behavior. Focus groups have been used successfully in a variety of settings. They are used in an exploratory manner to generate information about attitudes, opinions and hypotheses and to test new ideas. Focus groups are usually six to twelve members. The focus group is usually low cost, but the small group size makes it difficult to generalize findings to larger populations.

Community forum is less structured than other group assessments and can involve greater numbers of participants. Community forums are public meetings. They are useful for distributing information in a community, but can also generate initial feedback on topics presented to the community. The community forum allows all community members and groups to voice their opinions and concerns. The caution is to not let the forum degenerate into a gripe session.

Determining the Status of Existing Health Programs

Besides determining the health status of the target population, the status of health programs must also be determined. This also involves data collection methods similar to those already presented. Secondary data sources and primary data sources about the target population, the health care professionals and community leaders, can offer great insights and data to answer the following questions.

1. What are the programs and services available and accessible to the target population? Remember to examine all sources of services—public health organizations, community health organizations, volunteer organizations, religious organizations, etc.

2. What is the geographic proximity of the services to the population?

3. Are the programs and services utilized by the target population, and to what extent?

4. Are the programs and services meeting their organizational stated goals and objectives?

5. What is the actual cost of the service to the target population as consumers and to the taxpayer?

6. Are the services culturally appropriate and competent for the population(s) being served?

7. Are the needs of the target population being met? If not, why?

8. Are there available programs and services leading to positive changes in the quality of life for the target population?

9. Are there gaps in the services offered?

10. To what extent are services coordinated with other health and health-related services?

Analyzing the Data

Once the required data are collected, the health education specialist and the planning team must analyze the data to identify and prioritize problems and needs of the target population and those who will serve them. Due to limited funding and resources, setting priorities among the identified needs is warranted, since there are usually not enough resources to address all needs. After collecting the data, the health professional must analyze all of the data. The analysis of the data may be formal or informal. The formal analysis usually involves statistical analysis. The informal analysis which is used most often is commonly known as **eyeballing the data** (Windsor et. al., 1984). Eyeballing the data simply means looking at the data for differences between what exists and what ought to be. Again, the health education specialist must review and analyze the data according to the original plan of the needs assessment, answering the following questions.

- How can the target population be best described and defined?

- What is the current health status of the target population?

- What are the resources available to the community and target populations?

- How are the populations using the existing health services?

- What are the perceptions of the health providers regarding maternal, child and youth health needs?

- What are the perceptions of the community and the target populations regarding maternal, child, and youth health needs?

- Which variables, factors, indicators or precursors from the health system, providers, individuals, families, community and environment are identified as affecting the population's health status and the health system?

- Finally, define and describe the problems that the needs assessment has revealed to the planners.

Data analysis can be straightforward when there is agreement across all the data for a given issue. However, this may not be the case in situations in which the data for morbidity does not support the mortality data; or where the target population's perceptions of key health issues do not correspond with the data from the health care providers in the same community.

McKenzie et. al., (2013), suggest that using the first few phases of the PRECEDE PROCEED Model provides guidance in the problem analysis by answering the following questions:

1. Starting with Phase 1, what is the quality of life for the target population? Why did this group become the priority and focus of the needs assessment?

2. What are the actual and perceived social circumstances shared by those in the target population?

3. What are the social indicators in the target population that reflect these conditions (e.g., crime, absenteeism, school performance, poverty, unemployment, discrimination)? Do the statistical data support these findings?

4. Can the social conditions be linked to determinants of health addressed by health promotion?

5. Can these social conditions be linked to health problems? What are the health problems? How does the data support the linkage?

6. Which health problem(s) is most important for change and receives top priority for health education and health promotion efforts?

Problem Diagnosis

The sixth question is essential in identifying a prioritized list of problems and needs that the program plan will address. The planner must now complete the problem diagnosis. In examining the list of problems, the planner must have a clear understanding of which problems will set the direction and priorities for programs or interventions. This means that the planners must be able to identify the variables, factors, indicators and/ or precursors that relate to or cause the identified problem and impact health status. Given the identified problem, what are the social and health consequences of the health problem? The planner addresses the core variables of the identified problem through problem diagnosis. A systematic diagnosis of a health problem or need has four distinct stages: perception, verification, setting priorities, and analysis (Peoples-Sheps MD, et. al., 1996).

Perception

The perception of the problem is usually defined as the gap that exists between what is (the real) and what should be (the ideal). The perception of health problems must be addressed from the health education specialists' viewpoints and from the target populations' viewpoints. Ideally, if there is good communication among these groups and a strong working relationship, then there will not be great differences between the perceptions of needs for these groups. Therefore it is important to involve the target population throughout all phases of program development. The task of collecting data to determine this has been presented earlier. The need to collect data about suspected problems is to establish that the problem is not just someone's opinion or personal concern, but it is rooted in actual data. Indicators of health status and the ideal levels or the recommended levels for those indicators are required in diagnosing health problems and needs of the target population. The incidences of diseases or other health statistics are usually used as measures of health conditions. In other situations a variable or a risk factor may be highly predictive of a health problem, and will be measured in place of measuring the actual health problem or need. An example of this would be the measurement of incomplete DPT immunization status ". . . may be considered a surrogate indicator for a health problem, because a child who does not receive the full DPT series is at higher risk for diphtheria, pertussis, and tetanus than a child who receives the full immunization series"

(Peoples-Sheps MD, et. al., 1996). There are also situations when one risk factor contributes to several health conditions (e.g., smoking). Then using the risk factor as the focus for assessing multiple health status indicators may be efficient and productive.

In discussing problem perception, a word of caution is needed. It is most important not to define health problems as a service delivery deficiency. If this occurs, the planners are likely to focus on the lack of services or programs rather than a health problem. For an example, a health professional may observe that many of the high-risk prenatal clients bring their pre-school children to the clinic when they come for prenatal health care. Instead of the health care planners focusing on the health status of the prenatal clients and their real needs, they begin to plan child care or nursery services for the clients. While these services may be helpful, there is no evidence that the lack of child care service is a health problem for the target population. Kiritz (1980) refers to defining missing services as a problem as circular reasoning. The danger of this circular reasoning is that once the missing services are provided and the population participates in the services, the health care providers may declare that the problem is solved. However, the real problem has not been defined, because there is inadequate needs assessment. The needs for the pregnant women in this example are unmet. The focus of the development of health education and health promotion programs is to be responsive to the populations' health problems or unmet health needs, and not to spurious observations that have little to do with the real health needs of the population.

The health problem or unmet need has been defined as the difference between *what is* and *what should be.* The health education specialist's job is to determine the nature of the identified problem. When the true nature and context of the problem is determined, there may be many ways to intervene and many resources to be used. So problem diagnosis is essential to understand the problem, its characteristics, dynamics, its magnitude and severity, and its cause(s) or precursors. It is only when this diagnostic process is complete that the planners get clearer insights into how to effectively and efficiently address the defined problem(s).

Problem Verification

The verification process examines several aspects of the problems observed in the needs assessment to determine if the findings are really problems. The health education specialist must determine the extent of the identified problem(s), its duration, its expected future course and costs, and its variation across the community's population groups and geographic areas. Using the responses to the following questions, the health education specialist can verify that the identified problems are really problems for the target population:

1. What do you already know about the problem?
2. What information about the problem is missing?

3. Gather information on the problem—its causes and precursors, its characteristics, its incidence, its prevalence.

4. How many people are affected? What percentage of the total population do they represent?

5. How long has the problem been observed at the current level?

6. In what ways has the problem changed over time?

7. Clarify the definition(s) of the problem(s).

Setting Priorities

Public health and community health agencies are always faced with the dilemma of solving many health problems with limited resources: human, financial, or other resources. It becomes necessary to set priorities among problems and decide how to allocate limited resources to solving the problems. What must be the criteria for setting priorities for health problems? The criteria are not always straightforward because both the criteria and the problems may be controversial. It is not as simple as choosing problems that have serious consequences over those that have less serious consequences. Both types of problems may have controversial aspects. So in determining the criteria for prioritizing problems, it is important to have as much input from as many stakeholders as possible. The group of stakeholders should include representatives from the target population, state and local agencies, community organizations and businesses. It is essential that planners plan for equal and balanced input from all participants.

The following questions can indicate suggested criteria by which the program planner(s) may decide to set priorities among identified problems

1. Through the verification process, is the problem important? What is the pressing need?

2. Is it feasible to solve the problem? Are there adequate resources available to address the problem?

3. Are you the best people to solve the problem? Are others best suited to solve the problem? Who are they?

4. Have you weighed the positive and negative impacts of solving and not solving the problem?

5. Can the problem be solved in a reasonable time frame? Explain.

Problem Analysis

After completing the above process for identifying and prioritizing the health problems, the health education specialist and the planning committee should be ready to move forward to the final stage of problem analysis and developing a problem statement. According to Witkin and Altschuld (2000), there are many ways to analyze each problem. However, it is generally recommended that the planner consider a broad range of precursors and consequences that represent all domains of the problem

Figure 7.2 Problem diagram of low birthweight in Mercer County, Any State, USA

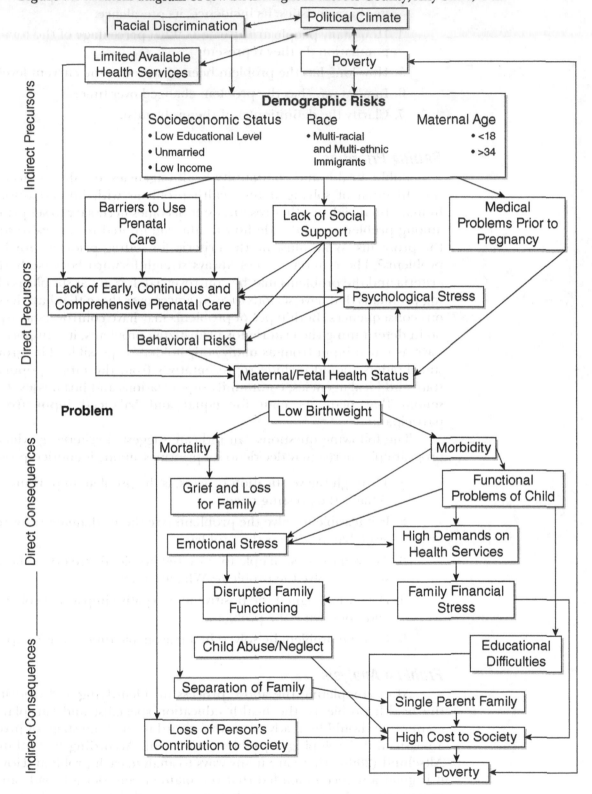

for the target population and health care providers. It would be helpful to diagram the problem and these domains to help conceptualize the problem and its various characteristics. Such a diagram could be helpful in the development of the program plan.

Peoples-Sheps et. al., (1996) suggests the use of a problem diagram. The problem diagram presented in Figure 7.2 has four components: the problem, the precursors to the problem, the consequences of the problem, and linkages. There is no real right or wrong way to illustrate these diagrams. The goal is to find the best way to demonstrate the precursors and consequences of a problem. In this diagram the problem appears in the middle of the diagram. The precursors are in the upper portion of the diagram and the consequences appear in the lower portion of the diagram. In both portions the precursors and the consequences are listed in the order of direct to secondary and to tertiary factors related to the problem. The arrows indicate the known and/or the hypothesized linkages. The precursors are factors associated with the problem. Some are directly linked and others are indirectly linked. The problem diagram presented here is for the hypothetical problem of low birthweight in Mercer County, AnyState, USA.

In the problem diagram, the precursors are the factors that influence, are strongly related to, and/or may be a cause of the problem of low birthweight. The consequences that appear in the diagram are the direct or indirect effects of the problem on the individual, family, and society. The health education specialist has learned about the precursors and consequences through the data collected in the needs assessment and through the professional literature and research generated about low birthweight.

It is important to note that the consequences of one cycle of the problem may become precursors of the next as indicated by the arrow connecting poverty in the consequences to the poverty in the precursor section. At the end of such a problem analysis, the health professional and others working as part of the planning team should have a clear conceptualization of the problem and all of the factors related to it.

The epidemiological and relative risk literature will help with the identification of the linkages. Relative risk is measured by an odds ratio, and is an indicator of the strength of the association between a risk factor and a health problem. This measurement is the ratio of the incidence of the problem in the population of people with the risk factor to the incidence in the population without the risk factor. Relative risk indicators can be used to identify risk factors for the problem diagram and to help determine the potential impact of intervening at a specific precursor. One example of this would be the comparative impacts of maternal smoking and maternal alcohol consumption. If maternal smoking has a higher relative risk for low birthweight than maternal alcohol consumption, then an intervention that is directed towards smoking cessation for pregnant women would potentially have more of an impact on low birthweight than an intervention that focuses on reducing alcohol consumption.

The Problem Statement

The health education specialist and the planning committee have completed the problem analysis. Now it is time to write the problem statement. The problem statement may be about two paragraphs in length and will include the following information:

- The defined condition, situation, or issue.

- Explain why the condition is sufficiently prevalent to be considered a problem?

- Which subgroups in the population are disproportionately affected by the problem? How are they affected?

- What is known about the relationships among precursors, consequences and the problem?

- Which of the direct and indirect precursors are more prevalent in the studied community compared to other communities?

- What are the precursors that the program will address to solve the problem?

- Which of the consequences will be relieved or eliminated as a result of reducing or eliminating the problem?

- Describe the target population who will be the focus of the program or intervention.

Reporting the Results of the Needs Assessment

The planners responsible for the needs assessment have completed the essential and initial tasks of the needs assessment. As a result of the needs assessment, the health problem(s) and/or issues have been identified and clearly defined. The results of the needs assessment should be shared with all members of the planning team, their administrators, the target population and its official representatives, other community stakeholders, as a formal report.

The health professional responsible for program development has completed the essential and initial tasks of the needs assessment of data collection and analysis. As a result of this process, the health problem(s) and/or issues have been identified. Next the planner must examine and clearly diagnose the problem(s), set priorities, develop a problem statement, develop the hypothesis for the recommended intervention, and develop realistic goals and objectives for the program.

References

Agency for Healthcare Research and Quality. 1995. *The Future of Children: Low Birthweight.* AHRQ Publication No. 00-P010. Rockville, MD. http://ahrq.gov/clinic/lobrhigh.htm.

Breckon, J., J. R. Harvey, and R. B. Lancaster. 1998. *Community Health Education: Settings, roles, and skills for the 21st Century.* Gaithersburg, MD: Aspen Publishers, Inc.

Butler, J. T. 2001. *Principles of Health Education and Health Promotion* (3rd ed.). Belmont, CA: Wadsworth/Thomas Learning.

Coreil, J., C. A. Bryant, and J. N. Henderson. 2001. *Social and Behavioral Foundations of Public Health.* Thousand Oaks, CA: Sage.

Cottrell, R. R., J. T. Girvan, and J. F. McKenzie. 2012. *Principles and Foundations of Health Promotion and Education.* Boston: Benjamin Cummings.

Doyle, E., and S. Ward. 2005. *The Process of Community Health Education and Promotion.* Long Grove, IL: Waveland Press, Inc.

Estes, G., and D. Zitow. 1980. *Heritage Consistency as a Consideration in Counseling Native Americans.* Paper read at the National Indian Education Association Convention, Dallas, TX.

Giger, J. N., and R. E. Davidhizar. 1995. *Transcultural Nursing Assessment and Intervention,* 2nd ed. St. Louis: Mosby-Year Book.

Joint Committee on Health Education and Promotion Terminology. (2012). Report of the 2011 Joint Committee on Health Education and Promotion Terminology. *American Journal of Health Education, 43* (2).

Kiritz, N. J. 1980. *Program Planning and proposal writing.* Los Angeles: The Grantsmanship Center.

McKenzie, J. F., B. L. Neiger, and R. Thackeray. 2013. *Planning, Implementing, and Evaluating Health Promotion Programs: A Primer.* Boston: Pearson Education.

Peoples-Sheps MD, A. Farel, and M. M. Rogers. 1996. *Assessment of Health Status Problems.* Washington, DC: Maternal and Child Health Bureau.

Simons-Morton, B. G., W. H. Greene, and N. H. Gottlieb. 1995. *Introduction to Health Education and Health Promotion.* Prospect Heights, IL: Waveland.

Specter, R. 2009. *Cultural Diversity in Health and Illness.* Upper Saddle River, NJ: Pearson/Prentice Hall.

Windsor, R., T. Baranowski, N. Clark, and G. Cutter. 1984. *Evaluation of Health Promotion and Education Programs.* Palo Alto, CA: Mayfield.

Witkin, R., and J. Altschuld. 2000. Planning and Conducting Needs Assessments. Thousand Oaks, CA, Sage. Yomiuri (2000).

Chapter 8

Health Education Process: Developing the Program Plan

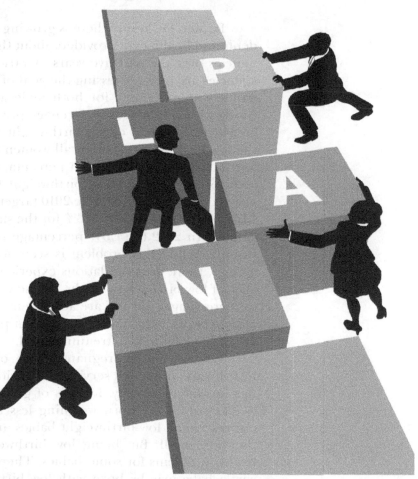

© Michael D. Brown, 2013, Used under license from Shutterstock, Inc.

Program planning is a complex process by which an intervention or program is designed to help meet the needs of a specific group of people, target population, or priority population. The health education specialist and the planning team will develop the hypothesis, goals, objectives, strategies in designing a program to meet the identified needs of the population that are identified in the needs assessment. The needs assessment produces a problem statement that is instrumental in developing a program plan. The contents of the problem statement are presented in the previous chapter. From the problem statement and other assessment findings the health education specialist should be able to produce a relevant and culturally appropriate program for the target population. See the example of a problem statement generated from the problem diagram presented in the previous chapter.

An Example of a Problem Statement for Low Birthweight Births in Mercer County

In Mercer County there is growing concern among its residents and health care providers about the increase in teen pregnancies over the past five years. A variety of health and social agencies are now addressing the goal of reducing teenage pregnancy with programs for both male and female adolescents. Along with this increase in teenage pregnancies, there is an increase in the births of low birthweight (LBW) babies. In 2008, the low birth weight rate for all women was 5.6% which was below the state low birthweight percentage of 6.8% in 2008. The goal for the state for low birthweight births was 5% by 2010, based on the Healthy People 2010 targets. However, by 2010, the LBW babies increased to 7.3% for the state and 9.7% for Mercer County. In 2012 the LBW percentage rose to 10.5% in Mercer County. While this problem is seen across racial and income groups, there are populations experiencing very high percentages of low birthweight births. Those who experience the highest percentages of LBW are adolescents 17 years old and under, members of newly arrived immigrant populations in urban areas of the county who are unmarried.

While teenage pregnancies are of great concern to the health care and social services professionals and the communities in Mercer County, LBW is of greater concern. Low birthweight babies are born weighing less than five pounds, eight ounces. Some low birthweight babies are healthy, even though they are small. But being low birthweight can cause serious health problems for some babies. There are two main reasons why a baby may be born with low birthweight: (1) premature births (babies born before 37 weeks of pregnancy; and Fetal growth restriction (small for gestational age). In the U. S. approximately seven of ten low-birthweight babies are premature. The earlier a baby is born, the lower the birthweight may be. About one in eight babies in the United States is born prematurely. Fetal growth restriction, the second reason for LBW births, results when the baby does not gain appropriate weight during the complete pregnancy.

The primary precursors for LBW births are lack of early, continuous and comprehensive care, psychological stress, behavioral risks (poor eating behaviors, poor nutrition, lack of personal hygiene, smoking) all of which impact on both the maternal and the fetal health status. The primary consequences of LBW are greater risks for infant mortality and morbidity that increase the emotional and economic stress for the mother, her family, and the infant. The consequences of LBW morbidity can continue and grow throughout childhood and adulthood.

The needs assessment reveals that the population experiencing the greatest percentage of LBW is a diverse population of recently arrived immigrants who are originally from eastern Europe, eastern Africa and Central America. Many of the population do not speak English. They do not know the health care system and especially do not seek prenatal care. The community is very low income with low literacy rates. Many cannot afford the costs of prenatal care so they do not seek it for pregnancy. Among those receiving care in the health clinics, there is adherence to traditional cultural practices that may be harmful to a developing fetus. For those teenagers who are pregnant and unmarried, shame may keep them from seeking care.

The Health Education and Health Promotion Committee for Healthy Pregnancies proposes a program to reduce low birthweight births in the city of Crawford in Mercer County. Such a program that will offer services to all pregnant women in Crawford will especially target pregnant adolescent and pregnant immigrant women, offering early prenatal care, education and support throughout their pregnancies and the first year of their babies' lives.

There are several good theories, models and frameworks that are useful in designing health education and health promotion programs. Some of these were presented in chapter six. There is no perfect model or framework that will accurately cover or predict all facets and outcomes of the program plan. However, every program design will include some specific components: the problem statement, the mission statement, the hypothesis, program goal(s), program objectives, program intervention methods, activities, an implementation plan and an evaluation plan.

Planning with People

The reader is reminded that the process of planning a health education program requires the contributions of the health education specialist as the planner, the target population, and other stakeholders in all aspects of the proposed program. The complexity of the planning process demands an organized and team approach to the process. This collaborative effort must allow representation and input from all who are involved in the decision-making. This will most often mean that the people and settings will be culturally diverse. Effective and collaborative work requires mutual respect for the diverse contributions and views of each member of the planning team and all of the stakeholders. The work of the planning group should result in the consensus of the group supporting a relevant program plan that truly meets the needs of all who are concerned.

Planning Assumptions

As the planning team designs a program to solve the health problem(s), it must consider the following assumptions that are characteristic of good planning. The overall assumption is that things do change in any environment.

- Factors in the external environment could affect the demand for the program. The planners must identify changing demographics in the target population and the community, new mandates, political changes, changes in services and resources that can affect the program plan and address them accordingly.

- Fiscal factors may change. Changes such as increased fees and funding cuts that may affect the program must be considered in the design of the program plan.

- There are consequences of all actions.

Planners must be able to predict the consequences of such changes. Examples of such planning assumptions are:

> The number of monolingual Spanish speaking families in the service area of the Rural Health Project is expected to increase by 30% over the next three years. Therefore culturally competent Spanish speaking administrative and health care staff must be hired to serve the population.

> The agency providing the educational materials used by the Rural Health Project will no longer produce the high quality promotional and health education brochures after this year because of funding cuts. Therefore the program must consider new suppliers of educational and promotional materials and the costs of such materials.

In these examples, the health education specialist would design the program's goals, objectives, methods, implementation, evaluation, and budgets to realistically consider the impact of these expected changes. The specifics of the assumptions are derived from the needs assessment.

The Hypothesis

As the health education specialist progresses through the needs assessment and problem analysis phases, it is clear that solving problems can be complicated. Before beginning any specific actions to address the defined problem(s), it is expected that the health education specialist first receive approval regarding the identified need and a mandate to proceed with the program design. The next step in designing the health program is formulating a hypothesis. Health issues and problems are complex and are often multifaceted, offering multiple opportunities and pathways to address a given problem. The health professional chooses a specific programmatic response to a health need based on (1) the logical determination of why the problem exists; (2) the understanding and application of the evidence-based literature; and (3) the application of appropriate theories, models, and/or frameworks in addressing changing health behaviors. The formulation of the hypothesis will link the problem analysis results to the proposed goals and objectives. "The hypothesis assures that there will be internal consistency among the program's components, and that the program can be evaluated" (Hanson, 1997, p. 7).

In the previous section, a sample health problem was presented for low birthweight births increasing in Mercer County. There are several precursors that are associated with the increase in the percentage of low birthweight babies being born in Mercer County (See the problem diagram on page 130 and the problem statement on page 138). The term precursor can also mean risk factor. The most direct precursors are maternal and fetal health status, behavioral risks, psychological stress, and the lack of early, continuous and comprehensive prenatal care. The behavioral risks include poor dietary pattern to support pregnancy, substance abuse, poor hygiene, risky sexual behavior during pregnancy and some cultural practices that may affect the pregnancy (pica consumption). At the secondary precursor level, the precursors are barriers to the use of prenatal care, the lack of social support, and medical problems prior to pregnancy. The primary and secondary precursors are generally impacted by availability of health services, poverty, discrimination, and the political climate controls the funds for available health services, but also has some relationship to the racial discrimination and poverty seen in Mercer County. The health education specialist examines these precursors or risk factors and links based on the most recent literature and the needs assessment data, and then determines which factors will be addressed by the program. The planners will want to choose those precursors or risk factors that will give the most powerful response and resolution to the problem.

In order to make the best choice of the precursors to address, the health education specialist ranks the factors by level of importance to the problem and changeability. The level of importance is how strongly the factor contributes to the problem: low, moderate, high. The changeability is the planner's determination of how likely the precursors and thus the problem, can be affected through intervention, given the available resources, political climate, individual and community responsiveness, etc. The program should be designed to address the most important and changeable factors that impact the problem the most for the target population.

Problem's Precursor/Risk Factor Analysis for Program Hypothesis

The following table has been constructed to help determine the level of importance and changeability of precursors or risk factors for the defined problem. The determination must be based on funding and other resources available to the planner as mandated by the employer or the agency's administration. The funding, the needs assessment results, and the most current analysis of the literature related to the problem and the target population are used in the determination of which problem precursors will be the focus of the program.

Problem: Increased LBW births among teen mothers ≤17 in Mercer County, Any State, USA.

The results of the precursor/risk factor analysis may have different responses to the importance and the likelihood of change from different health education specialists, based on their given target populations and the circumstances and resources of their communities and agencies.

Given the results of the analysis in Table 8.1, the precursors that are scored "high" as the most important to the problem and can most likely be changed through program interventions are:

- Behavioral risks (poor dietary pattern to support pregnancy, substance abuse, poor hygiene, risky sexual behavior during pregnancy and some cultural practices)

- Psychological stress

- Lack of early, continuous, and comprehensive prenatal care

- Barriers to the woman's use of prenatal care

- Lack of social support

The other factors are definitely important in reducing low birthweight births in Mercer County, but within the respective agency, the health education specialist may not have the means to make the greatest impact on the problem through these precursors. Through collaboration with other community agencies, stakeholders and resources the health education specialists may indeed be able to change these factors. For the purpose of this example for reducing low birthweight births, the focus will be on those precursors that scored high for both importance and changeability. The hypothesis will state what will happen to the health problem, if

Table 8.1 Precursor/Risk Factor Analysis for Program Planning

Precursors or Risk Factors Contributing to the Problem	Level of Importance (low, moderate, high)	Level of Changeability (low, moderate, high)
Maternal health status during pregnancy	High	Moderate
Fetal health status	High	Moderate
Behavioral risks (poor dietary pattern to support pregnancy, substance abuse, poor hygiene, risky sexual behavior during pregnancy and some cultural practices)	High	High
Psychological stress	High	High
Lack of early, continuous and comprehensive prenatal care	High	High
Barriers to woman's use of prenatal care (financial, language, transportation, cultural barriers)	High	High
Lack of social support	High	High
Medical problems before pregnancy	High	Moderate
Political climate	High	Moderate
Poverty	High	Low
Racial discrimination	High	High
Limited available health services (general health services for the general population)	High	Low

through effective and relevant programming the precursors can be reduced or eliminated. The hypothesis will also identify the consequences of such actions. The consequences will very likely be positive impacts and outcomes for the target population and the community. So based on the example's analysis, the hypothesis might be expressed as follows:

- If pregnant women with high risk behaviors improve their health status by adopting health behaviors relating to prenatal diet and nutrition, physical activity, substance use and abuse and risky sexual relationships in order to have healthy pregnancies and babies;

- If pregnant women adopted skills to reduce psychological stress during pregnancy and parenting;

- If early, continuous and comprehensive prenatal care are available for all pregnant women in Mercer County;

- If pregnant women in Mercer County can identify resources that enable them to overcome barriers to using of prenatal care (financial, language, transportation, cultural barriers);

- If pregnant women utilize social support resources in Mercer County

Then, the percentage of low birthweight births in Mercer County will decline to 5% by December 2015 with the following consequences:

- The barriers to women of all socioeconomic circumstances needing prenatal care will be reduced;

- There will be reduced infant mortality and morbidity rates in Mercer County among women receiving early, continuous and comprehensive health care;

- There will be improvement in the postnatal health status of the mothers and their children who received early and continuous prenatal care

The program hypothesis states the precursors that will be addressed or targeted in the program design in order to have the greatest impact on reducing the problem. The hypothesis also states the consequences or expected results of the program for the target population and the community. The hypothesis becomes the guide for developing the program plan and its components. It is important to note that in most of the precursors in our example health education will be appropriate, but it is also necessary to collaborate with other medical and social services to realize the decline in low birthweight births for Mercer county.

The Mission Statement

Most program plans begin with an overview or short narrative that describes the general purpose or direction of the proposed program. This narrative is usually referred to as a mission statement, program overview, program aim or statement of purpose. It gives the intent of the program and an indication of the philosophical perspective of the planning group that influences the goal(s), the objectives, the content and methods of the program. The health education specialist will be able to use the developed hypothesis in writing the mission statement, because the hypothesis does outline what the purpose or mission of the program will be.

Examples of mission statements

- The mission of the Women's HIV Prevention Program is to provide a range of services that will reduce the HIV infection rate among women of child-bearing age. It is expected that this program will result in the reduction of morbidity and mortality among women and children who are at risk, by preventing HIV infection.

- The Radiologic Services of Crawford City recognizes the importance of establishing and promoting healthy lifestyles among our employees. Healthy employees are productive and happy employees and citizens of this great city. This worksite health program will encourage employees at Radiologic Services to adopt healthy eating and physical activity behaviors to improve and maintain good health.

- Children are our most important resource in Mercer County. They must be cherished and protected from birth throughout life. The Mercer County Health Department understands that early, continuous and comprehensive prenatal care is a major investment in the lives of our citizens. This program, Upward Bound will provide the best start for our children through medical care and health education during pregnancy and into infancy.

Goals

Some health professionals use the terms **goals** and **objectives** as though they were the same, they are not the same. Goals are future events or outcomes toward which a given program or intervention is directed. Objectives are the steps that will be taken to reach or achieve the goal. Goals provide the destination, while objectives give us precise measurable directives to reach the destination.

Goals are general and broad statements of what will be achieved. Goals form the foundation for the program planning process. They must be clear and concise, and deal realistically with the problems and solutions of the target population (Butler, 2001). Goals are usually long-term, taking longer to complete than an objective. The goal(s) should be agreed upon by the planning group that is representative of all stakeholders.

Goals may or may not be written as complete sentences. Goals are often written in the infinitive verb form. Goals are usually not measurable by exact methods. There is no set number of goals that have to be stated in a program. Some programs will have only one goal while others will have several stated goals. In examining the developed hypothesis on reducing low birthweight births we have "if" and "then" statements. The "if" statements are the changes in the precursors or risk factors that will lead to the "then" statement. The "then" statement in the hypothesis becomes the program's goal.

Below are different ways the goal may be written.

The percentage of low birthweight births in Mercer County will decline

To reduce low birthweight births in Mercer County

To increase the number of full-term babies born at optimal birthweights

The goal statement usually includes:

1. Who or what will be affected?

2. What will change as a result of the program?

Other examples of goals.

- All cases of juvenile violence in Pico County schools will be eliminated

- To increase the consumption of fruits and vegetables among adult women in Barrett, USA.

- To reduce the incidence of HIV infection among women of child-bearing age

Objectives

As stated earlier, objectives are very specific and measurable steps that will lead to achieving goals. Objectives are smaller actions or steps that must be completed on the way to fulfilling or reaching a goal. Therefore they are crucial to any program plan, and much care must go into developing them and writing them. Objectives provide the health education specialist and other professionals with a clearer direction for achieving the change, impact, or outcome that will be accomplished in the program. Objectives make the selection of program strategies, methods and activities easier to choose. The selection of clear achievable and measurable objectives will also make program evaluation possible. Objectives should be written to address the most important and changeable factors. So in the low birthweight example, the 'If' statements that deal with the precursors or risk factors become the basis for objectives for the program's goal, if they are written in measurable terms. As the planners develop the objectives they must be sure that they also write objectives that can be measured in the evaluation process.

An example of a specific measurable objective in a program with the goal of reducing juvenile violence may have the following objective:

By the end of the academic year, 60% of students actively enrolled and participating in the program will demonstrate the basic skills for defusing potentially violent encounters.

The example illustrates the important elements that must be present in well-written objectives. Well-written objectives provide the planners with the means to not only select effective strategies and methods, but also the means for an effective evaluation process. McKenzie et. al., (2013, p. 143) provide the planners with these elements of the well-written objectives.

- The outcome to be achieved. (What will change?)

- The condition under which the outcome will be observed. (When will the change occur?)

- The criterion for deciding whether the outcome has been achieved. (How much change is proposed?)

- The priority population or the target population. (Who will change?)

The Outcome

The outcome is the first element and defines the status, action, behavior, or some other factor that will change as a result of the program. The outcome is usually the verb of the statement. So in the example, the outcome is reflected in the verb "demonstrate." The participants in this program will be expected to demonstrate very specific behaviors and skills: the basic skills for defusing potentially violent encounters. The demonstrated new knowledge and skills are assumed to lead to behavior that reduces violence in the schools. The verb "demonstrate" can be documented, so that the objective can be measured and evaluated. During the academic year how many students actually could "demonstrate" skills in defusing violent situations?

Listing of verbs related to cognitive, affective, and psychomotor domains can be helpful to the planner in writing objectives. The reader was introduced to the *The Bloom's Taxonomy of Educational Objectives* (Bloom, 1956), in Chapter 6. It has been instructive for educators for many years in finding appropriate verbs for specific and measurable objectives. Table 8.2 list a few verbs that can be used in objectives about changes in knowledge (cognitive domain), feelings and attitudes (affective domain), and skills and behaviors (psychomotor domain) that can be used for the outcome element in well-written objectives. These are verbs that relate to something that is measurable and observable.

Some verbs are not appropriate choices for outcomes because they cannot be measured nor observed. These would be verbs such as *know, appreciate,* and *understand,* which imply outcomes that cannot be measured, observed nor evaluated. So an example of a poor objective would be:

> By the end of the academic year 2015, 60% of students actively enrolled and participating in the program will understand the basic skills for defusing potentially violent encounters.

There is no way to measure objectively whether someone "understands" the basic skills, even if they perform them. "Understands" can mean different things to different people. More appropriate verb choices for our example might be *demonstrate, list, show,* or *illustrate* "basic skills for defusing potentially violent encounters."

The Condition

The "condition" relates to when the outcome will be observed. The condition is usually expressed in the objective as the date or time by when the outcome can be observed and measured. Some examples of terms and phrases that usually express the condition are "by the end of December 2003," "by June 30, 2004," "after completion of the training program," or "by the end of the class."

The Criterion

"The criterion" is the third element of the well-written objective. The criterion defines when the outcome is achieved, or how much change will

Table 8.2 Outcome Verbs for Objectives

1. *Knowledge:*	4. *Analysis:*	7. *Conveying Attitudes:*
define	analyze	acquire
describe	categorize	consider
identify	classify	exemplify
label	differentiate	modify
list	discriminate	plan
match	distinguish	realize
name	infer	reflect
reproduce	select	revise
select	separate	transfer
2. *Comprehension:*	5. *Synthesis:*	8. *Relating to Psychomotor:*
converting	compile	demonstrate
defend	compose	diagnose
describe	conclude	diagram
distinguish	create	empathize
estimate	design	hold
explain	explain	integrate
general	plan	internalize
interpret	propose	listen
paraphrase	revise	massage
predict	summarize	measure
	synthesize	operate
3. Application:		palpate
apply	6. Evaluating:	pass
change	appraise	prepare
compute	compare	project
discover	conclude	record
illustrate	contrast	visualize
modify use	describe	write
predict	evaluate	
prepare	explain	
produce	justify	
relate	summarize	
solve	support	

take place. It provides the standard by which the planners can decide if the outcome has been performed "in an appropriate and/or successful manner (McKenzie et. al., (2013)." In the earlier example of an objective, the phrase, "60% of students actively enrolled and participating in the program" tells the program planners and the program evaluators the standard for determining if the program is successful. Other examples of a criterion used in an objective are:

". . . 90% of women enrolled in prenatal services . . ."

". . . 80% of enrolled participants 19–24 years old . . ."

The Target

The target population is the fourth element that must be present in the well-written objective. This element tells who will change, such as "60% of *students actively enrolled and participating in the program.* The target population is not "students," but students who are enrolled and participating in the program. Other examples are "HIV+ women of child-bearing age in Pico County," "all infants born to women who are substance abusers," or "All employees of ACE Corporation."

The Hierarchy of Objectives

In order to achieve the goal(s) of a program, it is necessary to address different levels of objectives. Objectives are designed in a hierarchical manner, so that each objective at each level becomes successively more explicit. This means that the achievement of the lower level objectives contributes to the upper level objectives and the goal(s). Deeds (1992) offers a hierarchy of objectives and shows how each level relates to program outcomes, possible evaluation measures, and types of evaluation. The achievement of the lower level objectives will contribute to the achievement of the higher level objectives and goals (McKenzie et. al., 2013).

//

Hierarchy of Objectives and Their Relation to Evaluation

Level 1—Process or Administrative Objectives

The process or administrative objectives are the first level of objectives and include the daily activities and tasks that will lead to the accomplishment of other levels of objectives. These are the objectives that deal with all program details that shape the program: program resources, the appropriateness of intervention activities, recruitment regimen for the target population, program participation, attendance, feedback from program participants and other stakeholders, data collection methods, etc.

Examples:

- By June 30, 2015, 250 youth aged 12–16 will be recruited to the program.

- Two culturally appropriate brochures will be published for the African American participants' nutritional needs by December 31, 2015.

Level 2—Impact Objectives

The impact objectives are the second level of objectives. Impact objectives include three different types of objectives: learning objectives, behavioral objectives, and environmental objectives. These objectives are called impact objectives because they reflect the immediate observable effects of the program. They will show changes in awareness, knowledge, attitudes, skills, behaviors, or the environment. These objectives provide the foundation for the impact evaluation.

Learning Objectives

Learning objectives are the educational or learning tools that are needed in order to achieve the planned behavior change. Learning objectives relate to the predisposing, reinforcing, and enabling factors related to change. The learning objectives have their own hierarchy of four different types of learning objectives, moving from the least complex to the most complex. The level of complexity relates to time, effort, and resources necessary to accomplish the learning objectives. The levels for the learning objectives are also related to the learning domains.

1. Awareness objectives (the least complex)
2. Knowledge objectives (relates to the cognitive domain)
3. Attitudes objectives (relates to the affective domain)
4. Skills development or acquisition objectives (relates to the psychomotor domain)

Examine the following learning objectives and determine which of the learning objectives address awareness, knowledge, attitudes, and skill development.

1. _AS_ By the end of the academic year, 2016, 60% of students actively enrolled and participating in the program will demonstrate the basic skills for defusing potentially violent encounters.

2. _IA_ After the participants have examined the program brochure on type 2 diabetes; at least 40% will be able to identify all of the risk factors for type 2 diabetes.

3. _2K_ By the end of the class, 50% of pregnant participants will be able to explain the importance of iron in the diet during pregnancy.

4. _3K_ At the end of the program, 80% of the adolescent participants will debate their views of the pros and cons of teenage pregnancy.

Answers:

1. skill development
2. awareness
3. knowledge
4. attitude

Behavioral Objectives

Behavioral objectives are based on specific health behaviors that are linked to the identified health problem. Through the problem analysis the planners should have recognized target behaviors that are part of the cause, and effect relationship between the behavior and health issue. These objectives describe the behaviors or actions in which the target population will engage that will resolve the health problem and move toward achieving the program goal. The learning objectives that cover the cognitive, affective, psychomotor domains are written to support the fulfillment of behavioral objectives.

Examples of the behavioral objectives:

- One year after the completion of the program, 75% of the program participants who completed the Heart Health course will report having their blood pressure measured during the previous six months.

- Six months after the completion of the Diabetes Prevention Program, 70% of the participants completing 90% of the physical activity classes will follow a personal activity regimen for 20 minutes of vigorous activity for each of five days per week.

Environmental Objectives

Environmental objectives address the non-behavioral causes or precursors of or links to health problems that are identified from the needs assessment. The environmental changes may be defined as the physical, social, psychological, or cultural environments.

Example:

- By 2015, 75% of those without health care in Pico County will enroll in a health insurance plan that gives them access to quality health care.

- By 2016, 90% of the low-income communities in Potts City will have access to recreation centers, parks and walking trails.

Level 3—Outcome Objectives

Outcome objectives, also referred to as program objectives, state the ultimate end result or objectives of the program. They are objectives that are "outcome or future-oriented" that deal with changes in quality of life, health status, or social benefits (McKenzie et. al., 2013). The outcome objectives are usually written about reductions in risk, mortality, morbidity disability, or quality of life measures. When the outcome objective is accomplished, then the program goal is accomplished.

The success of a program will depend on the selection and specificity of the objectives for solving the problem. All of the levels of objectives should be included in a well-written program plan. This allows for greater opportunities to reach success in a variety of areas that directly relate to the program goal. So be sure to include objectives that are process objectives, impact objectives that include learning objectives, behavioral objectives, and environmental objectives, and outcome objectives in the program plan. Most importantly, the objectives and the methods that will be chosen for these objectives must be based on and affect the predisposing, enabling, and reinforcing factors which influence health behaviors and health status. These factors may also be expressed as precursors or risk factors. Every objective must be a SMART objective: SMART stands for specific, measurable, achievable , realistic, and time phased (CDC, 2003).

Program Interventions and Activities

After selecting the goals and objectives, planners must identify the strategy or intervention that leads to the achievement of the goals and objectives. The intervention is the planned method and activity or set of methods and activities that permit the most effective pathway to accomplishing the program goals and objectives, and the most efficient and responsible use of resources. The planning team may be temporarily expanded to include individuals or consultants with special expertise in policy development, educational methods, application of theory, and/or community organization. This allows the team to examine the variety of methods available and then choose the best methods for fulfilling each objective and reaching the program goal.

Methods are considered the general descriptions of how the change within the target population will be accomplished. In health promotion, methods may include community advocacy and development, communications and mass media, educational and instructional methods, counseling and behavior modification, group work, support groups, legislative and regulatory methods, policy development, environmental changes, health status appraisals, etc. In health education the methods are educational methods to change behavior based in learning principles and behavioral theories and models. Various methods will also include activities. The activities are specific events or opportunities used to execute the method and achieve the expected outcome of the objectives. The decision about the most effective and efficient methods and activities is central to the success of the program. Therefore, members of the target population must be consulted and included in the selection of intervention methods and activities. The inclusion of representatives of the target population can ensure that the methods and activities are educationally, culturally and socially relevant and appropriate.

There is abundant literature on various methods and activities that have been used in health promotion programs, and the theories and models upon which they are based. The decision for the best methods and activities must be based on sound rationale. While there is no perfect way to choose a successful method or intervention, the choice has to be more than "chance," "a good feeling" or "sounds good."

Table 8.3 lists some of the more popular and common methods used in health education to accomplish program objectives and program goals.

Table 8.3 Listing of Health Education Methods

Getting acquainted/icebreakers	Models
Audio	Music
Audiovisual materials	Newsletters/flyers
Brainstorming	Panels
Case studies	Peer education
Cooperative learning and group work	Personal improvement projects
Computer-assisted instruction	Problem solving
Debates	Puppets
Displays & bulletin boards	Role plays
Educational game	Self-appraisals
Experiments and demonstrations	Simulations
Field trips	Social media
Guest speakers	Storytelling and literary venues
Guided imagery	Theater (using scripts)
Humor	Value clarification
Lecture	Video conferencing
Mass media	Word games and puzzles

McKenzie and Smeltzer (1997) recommend some major considerations in creating a health promotion intervention. The following questions may serve as criteria for the selection of appropriate methods and activities.

- Are the selected methods based upon appropriate theory?

- Do the program methods and activities fit the goals and objectives of the program?

- Are the necessary resources available to implement the selected intervention, methods and activities?

- Are the interventions appropriate for the segmented target audience?

- What types of intervention methods and activities are known to be effective (successful in previous programs and with similar populations) in dealing with the program focus? Are the selection of methods and activities informed by evidence based practice and research?

- Would it be better to use an intervention that consists of a single event or one that is made up of multiple events and activities?

The responses to the questions can help to choose appropriate interventions. Some of the considerations in choosing intervention types appear in the flow chart for creating interventions.

Figure 8.1. Choosing the intervention type

Items to Consider when Creating a Health Promotion Intervention

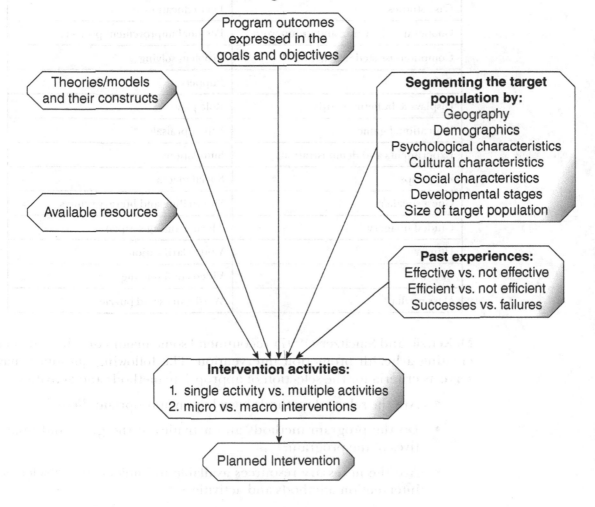

Program outcomes expressed in the goals and objectives

Theories/models and their constructs

Available resources

Segmenting the target population by:
Geography
Demographics
Psychological characteristics
Cultural characteristics
Social characteristics
Developmental stages
Size of target population

Past experiences:
Effective vs. not effective
Efficient vs. not efficient
Successes vs. failures

Intervention activities:
1. single activity vs. multiple activities
2. micro vs. macro interventions

Planned Intervention

References

Butler, J. T. 2001. *Principles of Health Education and Health Promotion,* 3rd ed. Belmont, CA: Wadsworth/Thomas Learning.

Doyle, E., and S. Ward. 2005. *The Process of Community Health Education and Promotion.* Long Grove, IL: Waveland Press, Inc.

Hanson, M. (Ed.). 1997. *Maternal and Child Health Program Design and Development: From the Ground Up; Collaboration and Partnership.* US Department of Health and Human Services, Maternal and Child Health Services.

McKenzie J. F., and J. L. Smeltzer. 1997. *Planning, Implementing and Evaluating Health Promotion Programs: A Primer,* 2nd ed. Boston: Allyn and Bacon.

McKenzie, J. F., B. L. Neiger, and R. Thackeray. 2013. *Planning, Implementing, and Evaluating Health Promotion Programs: A Primer.* Boston: Pearson Education.

Peoples-Sheps MD, A. Farel, and M. M. Rogers. 1996. *Assessment of Health Status Problems.* Washington, DC: Maternal and Child Health Bureau

Chapter 9

Health Education Process: Planning for Implementation

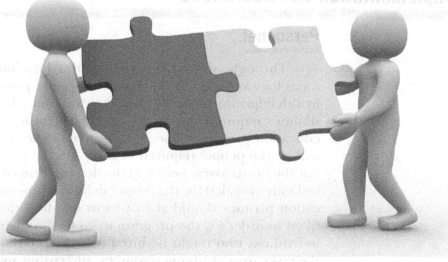

© Liviu Ionut Pantelimon, 2013. Used under license from Shutterstock, Inc.

The planner through the health education process has designed the various components of the program plan that is to be delivered to the target population. After the planning of the program comes the implementation of the program. Generally, implementation means the activation of the program plan. The implementation determines if the planners will be successful in producing the measurable changes, impacts and outcomes identified in the plan's objectives. The details and logistics of implementing a program will differ given the nature and scope of the program, the target population's characteristics, the number and the nature of cooperating organizations involved, the types of personnel to be recruited, hired and trained, needed facilities and equipment, other resources, and constraints. The implementation must be well planned and the roles of all stakeholders, professionals, and organizations clearly delineated. An implementation plan must also provide for appropriate funding and training needs.

Health education specialists must apply a variety of competencies and sub-competencies when fulfilling the responsibility of implementing the program plan. These include, but are not limited to, curriculum development, presentation skills, group facilitation skills, data collection as well as technology utilization (Cottrell et. al., 2012).

Implementation requires the health education specialist and the planning team to decide on the appropriate course of action for implementation, to write and execute clear and concise policy statement(s), and implementation plan. The health education specialist will continue to review and examine the role of cultural, social, ethnic, religious, spiritual, and behavioral factors in determining how the program is delivered. The planning team and the health education staff implementing the program will adhere to the code of ethics for health education professionals.

Implementation Considerations

Personnel

Throughout this book, the health education specialist has been the focus for carrying out the health education process. Needless to say, the health education specialist will not carry out all of the duties and responsibilities required for designing, implementing, and evaluating a health education program. The key resource of the health education program will be the people required to carry out the program services. Throughout the needs assessment and the development of the program plan many tasks are revealed for the proper delivery of the program. The health education planner should at first focus on all of the tasks that must be fulfilled in order for the program to go forth rather than trying to think of individuals who might be hired into the program prematurely. Some of the tasks are identifying resources, advertising, marketing, conducting the program, providing support services, services for those with disabilities, translating services with language challenges, evaluating the program, managing data, recordkeeping, budgeting, administrative tasks, etc. After creating the tasks lists, the health education specialist and the planning team can study existing and potential program resources. The planning team will now determine the appropriate positions to fulfill the identified tasks. The planners have internal personnel who are those individuals already working for the agency that is home to the program or they are members of the target population. Sometimes workers in other agency departments will change positions to work in a program after receiving appropriate training. On occasion there may be a need for a worker with certain specialized skills and there is a person in the target population who has that skill. The agency may have student interns from the local university willing to serve in the program or there may be peer educators from the local high school willing to work with other children or youth. The other source of personnel is external or outside of the home planning agency. These may be people outside of the agency who would conduct all or part of the required services. These individuals may only fill in the "gaps" that cannot be filled within the home agency. Others will be hired for a specific position to fulfill tasks. The agency may contract with an outside vendor for a person or persons to provide services to the program. Regardless of the planner's choice, appropriate training for the specific program tasks and services is required in preparation for the program's start.

Fiscal Planning and Budgeting

Program implementation must necessarily include fiscal planning and budgeting. This will assure that appropriate funds and resources are properly matched with fiscal needs and demands. A budgeting process is required to be sure that limited resources are not wasted and that overexpenditures do not occur. The costs of resources that include personnel, materials, equipment, and the program site can make or break the planned program. If the health education specialist is responsible for implementing a program plan that does not have adequate financial resources, then he or she may also be responsible for securing the funds to support the program. This may be done through the health education specialist seeking donations or sponsors, through grant sources, or fundraising events. How funds are secured for health programming will depend on the agencies' policies and directives. Health education specialist will follow agency protocol in all aspects of implementation. If the health education specialist receives permission to seek donations, be sure that other divisions in the agency are not requesting funds from the same companies or sponsors. Corporate sponsors usually pay for the costs of a program that it is interested in or a portion of that program. There is no single way to seek corporate funding. Often contact is made with a potential donor with a letter, a face-to-face meeting or a telephone call. Again, be certain that the funds that they will donate can be accepted by the planner and the agency. The health professional will not overwhelm a donor with excessive requests.

Grant funding is a very common way to secure funds. There are a great number of federal, state, and local government agencies that offer money for health programs. Funding is also offered for health programs by many voluntary agencies (i.e., American Heart Association, the American Cancer Society, etc.), foundations, and professional organizations. There are even private individuals who offer funds to support health programming in which they are interested. It is strongly suggested that health education specialists spend time on the internet and identify the many agencies that would provide grant funding for a specific health program. In most cases grant funding begins with an application completed by the appropriate agency official and submitted to the funding organization. Most of these organizations will request a program proposal. Grant proposal writing has much in common with the process of developing a program plan. The program plan can inform the grant writing. The main difference in the two is that the grant proposal is usually a strongly competitive process. The funding of the program plan will depend on how well the planner can write the proposal so that it will be chosen for funds above all other proposals submitted to the funding organization. Doyle and Ward (1997, p. 176) share tips for successful grant proposals.

The successful grant proposal:

- Perfectly adheres to the funder's requirements.

- Will be based on an innovative idea. Even if it is an old idea put in a new and innovative package.

- Will advance the practice of health education and/or community health.

- Will fill a critical gap in knowledge.

- Will be driven by sound evidence, theory, and research.

- Works toward a long-term goal.

- Includes a thoughtful and up-to-date literature review.

- Is well-written.

- Provides evidence of feasibility.

- Demonstrates an appropriate choice of methods.

- Is well-focused.

- Has a well-thought out evaluation plan.

Pilot-Testing, Phasing in, and Total Implementation

Health education specialists will plan the implementation of a program based on available resources and the setting for which the program is intended. However, it is important to consider three critical factors that contribute to the success of health program plans. Health promotion programs work well when the implementation addresses the following:

1. The recipients are recognized, respected, and treated as contributors throughout the planning, implementation, and evaluation of the program.
2. Those responsible for delivering the program are qualified and competent.
3. There is responsible evaluation and reporting of the program's impacts and outcomes.

Three major ways of implementing a program are suggested by Parkinson et. al., (1982): pilot testing, phasing-in, and initiating the total program.

Pilot-Testing

Pilot testing (piloting or field testing) a program permits the health education specialist and staff to implement the program on a small scale with a small number of the target population. Pilot testing allows the planners to have close control of the program. It enables the planners to identify and solve any problems that may exist before the program is offered to a larger number of the target population. Ideally the pilot testing should occur with people who are like the target population and in a similar setting. Planners will want to be sure that:

1. staff selection and training are adequate and appropriate.
2. planned methods and activities work.
3. program is marketed appropriately.
4. facilities are appropriate.
5. program timelines, schedules, and logistics are worked out.
6. program participants are given the opportunity to evaluate the program.

The evaluation of the program by the participants is part of process evaluation or formative evaluation. The participants are able to evaluate program content, methods and activities, practitioner or instructor effectiveness, facilities and space, accommodations, etc. As a result of the process feedback, planners will make changes in the program. If many changes are made, it may be necessary to pilot test the program again.

Phasing In

When there is a very large target population, pilot testing should be followed by the phasing in of the program rather than implementing the full program. Phasing in the program allows the planner to have greater control over the program. It helps to prevent planners and program staff from being overwhelmed. Phasing in the program can be done by setting up various stages by using the following techniques to control the number of participants coming into the program:

1. limiting the number of participants from the target group entering the program at one time; set up intervals for admissions.
2. choice of location or setting; time the start of programs in different settings, so they do not all begin at once.
3. addressing a particular skill level of the participants; instead of bringing all residents in a setting into the program. For a community project that serves everyone in a given location, it may be more manageable to begin with parents first, then adolescents and then the children ten and younger.
4. offering particular aspects of the program activities. Instead of offering the whole program to a population, some participants could begin with one program feature while others begin a different program feature. Eventually all participants will participate in all offerings, but not all at one time.

Example:

If Pico County Health Department wanted to phase in their planned HIV Prevention Program for women of childbearing age, the planners might do the following things to phase in the program.

1. Limiting the number of participants from the target group.
   The implementation of the program will be focused on adolescents and young adults. With each new quarter of the year, services for a new age group will be added.

2. Choice of location or setting.
   The program is implemented only in the northwest part of the county for the first four months. The next four months of the program services will be offered in the northwest part of the county and in the southeast part of the county. Every four months, a new part of the county is added until the total county is receiving the program services.

3. Addressing a particular skill level of the participants.
   If the program included activities for increasing physical activity levels, the planners might start with beginning exercisers. Then in three months add services for intermediate exercisers. Finally, services would be added for advanced exercisers.

4. Offering particular aspects of the program activities.
   Planners may decide to begin program services with classes in stress management, and then add assertiveness training.

Total Implementation

Seldom would total implementation be appropriate without the pilot testing and phasing in processes. Pilot testing and phasing in will lead to necessary revisions in the program and the resolution of identified problems in the program's implementation. Total implementation can only benefit significantly from the pilot-testing and the phasing in. However, in some instances, only total implementation is possible. Programs that are planned or implemented around a single event, such as a lecture, screening event, or a one day health fair are exceptions; the health education specialist would offer the total program all at once for these types of events.

Other Concerns

Informed Consent

The well-being of the program participants is of primary concern. Every participant must be fully informed about the benefits and the risks of participating in the program. Informed consent from the participant is a requirement for any individual participating in any health promotion program. McKenzie et. al., (2013) suggest that program facilitators prepare participants for obtaining informed consent by doing the following:

1. Explain the nature and purpose of the program.
2. Inform program participants of any inherent risks or dangers associated with participation and any possible discomfort they may experience.
3. Explain the expected benefits of participation.
4. Inform participants of alternative programs or procedures that will accomplish the same thing.
5. Indicate to the participants that they are free to discontinue participation at any time.

Health education specialists must know that the participant's signing of the informed consent documents is not a release of liability or waiver of liability. If the health education specialist or any program staff person is negligent they can be found liable.

Policies and Procedures

The health education specialist and the program staff will address how the program moves toward the fulfillment of its goals and objectives through specific written policies and procedures. These will need regular review and updating in order to be relevant for the target population(s) and the program personnel delivering the services. Careful thought and preparation should be involved in policy development. Who will have the responsibility for developing policies and procedures? Who will administer the policies? Who in the agency will approve and oversee the policies and procedures?

Timeline

A tentative timetable can be very helpful in keeping the health education specialist and the program staff on task for program implementation. Such a timetable can be useful for all of the planning and implementation processes. Below is an example of a planning and implementation timetable. Every responsibility of the planners and the program staff must be scheduled and that schedule must guide the development and implementation of the program. Those who are responsible for the planning and implementation might prefer a more detailed schedule or calendar and for a longer period of time, if required.

Reporting

Planners will need to document and report the ongoing progress of the program to the target population, other stakeholders, administrators, and the community. The documentation and reporting is vitally important (1) for keeping the current participants motivated; (2) for recruiting new participants; (3) for public relations and for keeping the community involved; (4) for accountability.

Sample Timeline for Planning, Implementation, and Evaluation

Programming Tasks Year 1	Responsible Personnel	JAN	FEB	MAR	APR	MAY	JUN	JUL	AUG	SEP	OCT	NOV	DEC
Assemble the planning committee.	Project Director	X											
Conduct the needs assessment.	Planning Committee		X	X									
Develop hypothesis, goals, and objectives.	Planning Committee				X	X							
Review policies and rules.	Planning Committee				X	X							
Design intervention/methods/activities.	Project Staff						X	X					
Assemble resources.	Project Manager						X	X					
Market the program.	Project Staff & Planning Committee									X	X		
Recruit program participants.	Project Staff									X	X		
Pilot test program.	Nurses and Health Educators											X	X
Process evaluation.	Project evaluator and staff											X	X

Programming Tasks Year 2	Responsible Personnel	JAN	FEB	MAR	APR	MAY	JUN	JUL	AUG	SEP	OCT	NOV	DEC
Review and revise the program.	Project Staff	X	X										
Market the program.	Project staff & Planning Committee			X	X								
Recruit program participants.	Project staff			X	X								
Phase in Part 1.	Nurses & Health Educators					X	X						
Phase in Part 2.	Nurses & Health Educators							X	X				
Total implementation.	Nurses & Health Educators									X	X		
Impact evaluation.	Project staff									X	X		
Prepare evaluation report.	Project Evaluator											X	
Distribute report.	Project Director												X

Cultural Competence

As mentioned in other places in this text, the health education specialists are urged to include responsible representatives of the target population and other stakeholders who are respected and trusted by the community. They must be involved throughout the planning, implementation, and evaluation stages of the program. To accomplish this and to be successful with the program, cultural competence is required. Cultural competence is based on the principle that all individuals are to be treated equally, respectfully, and are to receive the best and appropriate care regardless of race, ethnicity, culture, religion, or creed. The health education specialist, the planning team, and the program staff must demonstrate cultural competency throughout the planning, implementation, and evaluation of the program. It may be the responsibility of the health education specialist to train the program staff in cultural competence. It is important that the staff treat all persons, even their fellow workers with respect, honoring each person for who he or she is and what they bring to the program. All persons should receive the same respect and quality of service and communication in the program operations. This is not a matter of race or color because culture is so much more than that. The goal of offering quality health care to all people must be the focus and how to overcome barriers to the access to quality health services.

The Office of Minority Health, US Department of Health and Human Services offers this reminder about the importance of cultural competence in health professionals:

> . . . It's the way patients and doctors can come together and talk about health concerns without cultural differences hindering the conversation, but enhancing it. Quite simply, health care services that are respectful of and responsive to the health beliefs, practices and cultural and linguistic needs of diverse patients can help bring about positive health outcomes. (OMH, 2013)

The implementation plan must include a marketing plan to reach the target population with an outreach system and messaging that is respectful, ethical and addresses the cultural sensitivities of the target population. The program offered must be of the highest quality given the program resources to achieve program goals and objectives.

References

Butler, J. T. 2001. *Principles of Health Education and Health Promotion,* 3rd ed. Belmont, CA: Wadsworth/Thomas Learning.

Doyle, E., and S. Ward. 2005. *The Process of Community Health Education and Promotion.* Long Grove, IL: Waveland Press, Inc.

Huff, R. M., and M. V. Kline. 1999. *Promoting Health in Multicultural Populations, a Handbook for Practitioners.* Thousand Oaks: Sage Publications.

McKenzie, J. F., B. L. Neiger, and R. Thackeray. 2013. *Planning, Implementing, and Evaluating Health Promotion Programs: A Primer.* Boston: Pearson Education.

Office of Minority Health. 2013. *What is Cultural Competency?* Retrieved on June 12, 2013 at http://www.minorityhealth.hhs.gov/templates/browse.aspx?lvl=2&lvlid=11.

Simons-Morton, B. G., W. H. Greene, and N. H. Gottlieb. 1995. *Introduction to Health Education and Health Promotion.* Prospect Heights, IL: Waveland.

Specter, R. 2009. *Cultural Diversity in Health and Illness.* Upper Saddle River, NJ: Pearson/Prentice Hall.

Chapter 10

Health Education Process: Planning for Program Evaluation

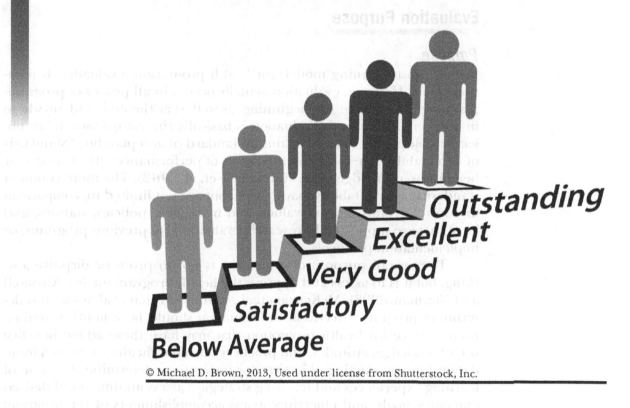

Outstanding

Excellent

Very Good

Satisfactory

Below Average

Program evaluation is crucial to health education and health promotion programming and serves many purposes. A plan for program evaluation is developed as the goals, objectives, and methods are developed for the program plan. If the objectives for changed behavior and health status are written correctly they will yield the measures needed to evaluate the program. Without well-written and SMART objectives there is no reliable program evaluation.

Evaluation unfortunately is often misunderstood. Butler (2001) identifies some of the reasons why evaluation is misunderstood. Students often view evaluation as a test for which they must cram to get a good grade. Health education specialists sometimes see evaluation as the laborious task of filling out forms that only result in meetings with supervisors to discuss their deficiencies. Supervisors, planners, and teachers may see evaluation as a way of enforcing discipline on employees and students. Evaluation is none of these. Program evaluation is none of these things.

Evaluation Purpose

Purpose

In most planning models for health promotion, evaluation is mentioned last. However, evaluation actually occurs in all phases of program-planning. It occurs at the beginning, as well as at the end, and anywhere in-between, if required. Evaluation is basically the comparison of an object or objective of interest against a standard of acceptability. "Standards of acceptability are the minimum levels of performance, effectiveness, or benefits used to judge value" (McKenzie et. al., 2013). The more common standards of acceptability may include, but are not limited to, comparison or control groups, norms, values, and mandates (policies, statutes, and laws) that are supported by research, evaluations of previous programs, or implementation protocols.

The overall purpose of evaluation is not to prove or disprove anything, but it is to assess and improve the health program quality (Creswell and Newman, 1993). McKenzie et. al., (2013) add that evaluation also determines program effectiveness. Evaluation should be a nonthreatening, positive force for health promotion that may have these added benefits: offer knowledge, attitudes, and practices related to health, serve as a foundation for constructing objectives for instruction; determine the value of learning experiences and teaching strategies; assess attainment of desired outcomes, goals, and objectives; assess accomplishments of the program; identify limitations or weaknesses of the program; assess the value of learning aids and materials and the ways in which they have been used; determine the level of achievement for each individual student/client, as well as for the group; and justify the program and its expenditures (Butler, 2001).

Elder et. al., (1994) describes evaluation as the systematic process of collecting and analyzing reliable and valid information at various points and processes in the program in order to improve program effectiveness, reduce costs and to contribute to future planning efforts. Program evaluation must always emphasize reliable, valid and systematic information and does not really differ in substance from "real" research. However, through its orientation toward quality enhancement, cost effectiveness, and planning, program evaluation may take on a much different tone than its epidemiological or clinical trial counterparts (Elder et. al., 1994). Thus evaluation must yield accurate information to determine the process, impact and outcome of health education and health promotion programs and health services. It also enables planners to make decisions based on accurate information and not on speculation.

Who Conducts the Evaluation?

Planners will have to determine who conducts the evaluation. Evaluators must avoid conflict of interest and be as objective as possible. The evaluator may be someone associated with the program or someone who is external to the program. The internal evaluator is someone who has the advantage of being closer to the program staff and activities, so the collection of relevant information is easier. The internal evaluator is less expensive usually than hiring additional staff to conduct the evaluation. The disadvantage of using the internal evaluator is the possibility of evaluator bias. Certainly someone involved in the program has an investment in its outcome.

The external evaluator is usually more objective, but also more expensive than the internal evaluator. The external evaluator of course has less experience with the program and should provide unbiased evaluation results. The program planners may find it helpful to employ consultants with evaluation expertise to develop the evaluation plan.

Writing Measurable Objectives for Program Evaluation

As stated earlier, goals are general statements about the proposed changes in health status and/or quality of life for a target or priority population. They give the future big picture of what the program plan will accomplish for the population. Goals provide a sense of where the planners and the population want to go, but they give us no specific steps on how to reach the destination.

Objectives are the measurable statements that will lead to the accomplishment of the program goals. Earlier the reader was instructed on how to write effective and measurable objectives. There are a variety of instructions from credible sources on how to write measurable objectives. The key is that the well-written objective is a clear directive on how to reach a program goal. Objectives are process objectives, impact objectives or outcome objectives. These then align themselves with the categories of evaluation in one framework: process evaluation, impact evaluation, and outcome evaluation (Green & Kreuter, 1991). The program planners must be sure to include the key elements in every objective: the outcome to be achieved (what will change); the condition under which the outcome will be observed (when will the change occur); the criterion for deciding whether the outcome has been achieved (how much change is proposed); and the priority population or the target population (who will change). The objective that is well-written serves to guide the program staff on the methods and activities that must be implemented effectively, what data must be collected and measured to determine if the objective has accomplished what was originally planned.

Presented here is an example of a program being developed by health education specialist Laura. She has developed the program's mission statement, program goal and objectives. Can you determine what kind of evaluation, process, impact, or outcome would be used for each objective?

///

In the Pico County Health Department, Laura is responsible for designing a series of HIV/AID Prevention workshops for women of childbearing age. She is working on the orientation workshop design and implementation and "Method 1: Health Appraisal." What would her evaluation plan include for this workshop and how will it fit in the overall evaluation plan that she should have for this program? The program's mission statement, goals, objectives, and some methods are offered here.

The Pico County Women's HIV Prevention Program

Mission Statement

The mission of the Pico County Women's HIV Prevention Program is to provide a range of services that will reduce the HIV infection rate among women of child-bearing age. It is expected that this program will result in the reduction of morbidity and mortality among women and children who are at risk, by preventing HIV infection.

Goal

To reduce the incidence of HIV infection among women of child-bearing age in Pico County.

Objectives

Outcome objective

By the end of the year 2020, there will be a 20% reduction in the incidence of HIV infection among the women of childbearing age in Pico County.

Impact objectives:

A. *Behavioral objectives*

1. By the end of the program, 60% of the women abusing drugs will terminate their drug abuse behavior.

2. By the end of the program, 60% of the program participants who have been involved in risky sexual behavior will terminate that behavior.

B. *Environmental objectives*

1. By the end of the program's first year, 50% of the churches in target communities will participate in recruiting women who are high risk for HIV infection, to the program through trained peer advisors in the churches.

2. By the end of the program's first year, 50% of the churches in the target communities will offer a program of support services to program participants in their communities, through trained peer advisors in the churches.

C. *Learning objectives*

1. Awareness Level

   At the end of the program orientation session, 85% of the women participating in the session will be able to identify their own risks for HIV infection.

2. Knowledge Level

   By October 31, 2016, 75% of the participants will explain how HIV is transmitted.

3. Attitude Level

   By the third session, the program participants will express their views on how women can best protect themselves from HIV infection.

4. Skill Development/Acquisition Level

   By the completion of the Pico County Women's HIV Prevention Program, 75% of the participants will be able to demonstrate at least two stress management methods taught to them, that they use to reduce stress in their lives.

Process objectives

1. By August 30, 2016, 250 women of child-bearing age who are at risk for HIV infection will participate in the Pico County Women's HIV Prevention Program.

2. By August 30, 2016, all learning materials and outreach materials will be culturally competent in design and content.

Intervention strategy (strategies) to meet these objectives

Method 1: Health status appraisal

Activity 1A: Each participant attends the Orientation Session. Each participant completes the health appraisal form during the program participants' orientation session. Each participant determines health risk factors. Discussion leader introduces each participant to the concepts of risk factors and protective factors and how they impact their health status.

Method 2: Counseling

Activity 2A: Each participant is assigned to a personal counselor who provides support and guidance as each participant develops a plan for behavior change, implements her plan, monitors and evaluates the changes and outcomes. Participant must meet with and work with her counselor at least once per week.

Method 3: Group work

Activity 3A: Each program participant is assigned to a support group of approximately 10 women participating in the program. The group meets once every two weeks to gain new information, learn and practice new skills that promote health, and to provide support and accountability.

How will Laura determine if she has achieved the objectives for the workshop and if the workshop actually makes a difference for her participants?

Evaluation Terminology

Laura has decided to use the evaluation framework that aligns with the categories of her objectives to guide her on how to plan the evaluation of her program. There are generally two sets of terminology used by authors addressing levels or types of evaluation. Some use the terms process, impact and outcome evaluation. While other authors use the terms diagnostic, formative and summative evaluation.

The first framework discussed here has three levels of evaluation (Green and Kreuter, 1991) and asks different questions about the program or activity, addresses different aspects of the program or its effects, and deals with different indicators. Process evaluation examines how well the program or activity being implemented relates to the actual program plan. Impact evaluation determines the changes that occur in the target population's knowledge, attitudes, beliefs, values, skills, behaviors, and practices as the result of the program or intervention. Impact evaluation also measures changes in policies, programs and resources at the organizational level. At the governmental level, impact evaluation may show changes in policies, plans, legislation and funding related to given issues. Outcome evaluation identifies the improvements in health or social factors as the result of the intervention. Outcome evaluation examines the health status of the target population, morbidity rates that are at issue, and mortality rates that are at issue. Figure 10.1 illustrates process, impact, and outcome evaluation and the types of data measured for each. The needs assessment is considered an important part of the evaluation process in this framework and is included in the diagram. The needs assessment provides much of the baseline data.

Figure 10.1 Process, impact, outcome, and related data measurements

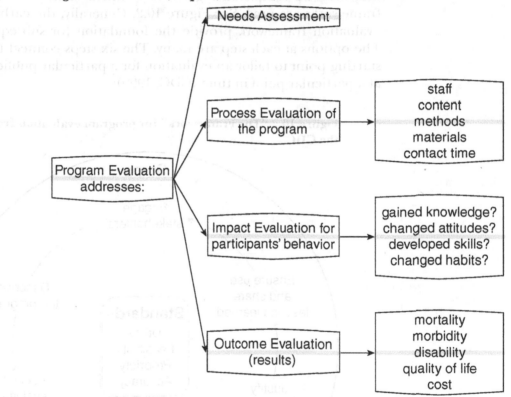

The second framework includes the terms diagnostic, formative and summative evaluation. Diagnostic evaluation is the needs assessment process. It commonly applies to individuals and groups to determine their needs for knowledge, attitude change, behavior change, or skill development. Formative evaluation begins when the program is being formed and continues throughout the program implementation to identify needed adjustments in the program. Formative evaluation is closely aligned with process evaluation. After the program is completed, the summative evaluation is implemented to examine all measurements and data that leads to judgments about the impact and outcomes of the program and to determine if the program should continue or to identify needed modifications prior to the program's next operation. Summative evaluation covers both impact and outcome evaluations discussed in the first evaluation framework.

Planning for the Evaluation Process

In 1999 the Centers for Disease Control and Prevention (CDC) published a framework for evaluation developed by a working group that includes public health officials, public health program experts and evaluation experts. This framework continues to be an important and an effective framework for evaluation. The framework has six stages or steps that must be completed regardless of which of the first two evaluation frameworks are used. See Figure 10.2. Generally, the earlier steps in the evaluation framework provide the foundation for subsequent progress. The options at each step are many. The six steps connect to be used as a starting point to tailor an evaluation for a particular public health effort, at a particular point in time (CDC, 1999):

Figure 10.2 "The Framework" for program evaluation from the CDC

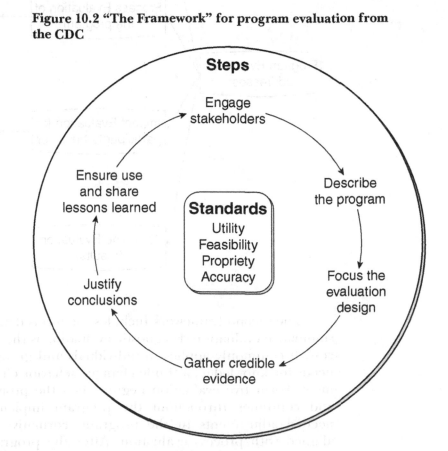

Steps

Engage stakeholders

Ensure use and share lessons learned

Describe the program

Standards
Utility
Feasibility
Propriety
Accuracy

Justify conclusions

Focus the evaluation design

Gather credible evidence

1. Engage stakeholders, including those involved in program operations; those served or affected by the program; and primary users of the evaluation.

2. Describe the program, including the need, expected effects, activities, resources, stage, context and logic model.

3. Focus the evaluation design to assess the issues of greatest concern to stakeholders while using time and resources as efficiently as possible. Consider the purpose, users, uses, questions, methods, and agreements.

4. Gather credible evidence to strengthen evaluation judgments and the recommendations that follow. These aspects of evidence gathering typically affect perceptions of credibility: indicators, sources, quality, quantity, and logistics.

5. Justify conclusions by linking them to the evidence gathered and judging them against agreed-upon values or standards set by the stakeholders. Justify conclusions on the basis of evidence using these five elements: standards, analysis/synthesis, interpretation, judgment, and recommendations.

6. Ensure use and share lessons learned with these steps: design, preparation, feedback, follow-up, and dissemination.

The CDC then ask the professional to apply the 30 standards of "The Framework." The standards are distributed into four groups of evaluation standards as a "lens" to help isolate the best approaches at each step. The 30 standards assess the quality of evaluation activities, determining whether a set of evaluative activities are well-designed and working to their potential.

The evaluation standards groups are:

1. Utility standards ensure that an evaluation will serve the information needs of intended users.

2. Feasibility standards ensure that an evaluation will be realistic, prudent, diplomatic, and frugal.

3. Propriety standards ensure that an evaluation will be conducted legally, ethically and with due regard for the welfare of those involved in the evaluation, as well as those affected by its results.

4. Accuracy standards ensure that an evaluation will reveal and convey technically adequate information about the features that determine worth or merit of the program being evaluated.

Reporting The Evaluation Results

The program evaluator must generate a final report that includes the data analyses, interpretation, and results to the stakeholders. Usually the number and types of reports are decided at the beginning of the evaluation based on the needs of the stakeholders. The evaluation reports must be timely to achieve important program improvements. The program evaluator must write the report and/or deliver the report orally so that it is communicated to all audiences.

The format of the evaluation report is similar to that used for research reports. McKenzie et. al., (2013) offer a description of the evaluation report, as summarized in Table 10.1.

Table 10.1 Format for an Evaluation Report

Abstract/executive summary	Overview of the program and evaluation. General results, conclusions, and recommendations.
Introduction	Purpose of the evaluation. Program and participant description (including staff, materials, activities, procedures, etc.). Goals and objectives. Evaluation questions.
Methods/procedures	Design of the evaluation. Target population. Instrument Sampling procedures. Data collection procedures. Pilot study results. Validity and reliability. Limitations. Data analyses procedures.
Results	Description of findings from data analyses. Answers to evaluation questions. Addresses any special concerns. Explanation of findings. Charts and graphs of findings.
Conclusions/ recommendations	Interpretation of results. Conclusions about program effectiveness. Program recommendations. Determining if additional information is needed.

References

Butler, J. T. 2001. *Principles of Health Education and Health Promotion,* 3rd ed. Belmont, CA: Wadsworth/Thomas Learning.

Centers for Disease Control and Prevention. 1999. *Evaluation Steps.* Retrieved on June 11, 2013 at http://www.cdc.gov/eval/steps /index.htm.

Centers for Disease Control and Prevention. 1999. "Framework for Program Evaluation in Public Health." *MMWR* 48 (No. RR-11): 1–40.

Creswell, Jr., W. H. and I. M. Newman. 1993. *School Health Practice (10th edition).* St. Louis: Times Mirror/Mosby.

Doyle, E., and S. Ward. 2005. *The Process of Community Health Education and Promotion.* Long Grove, IL: Waveland Press, Inc.

Elder, J. P., S. A. McGraw, and E. J. Stone, et al. 1994. "Catch-Process Evaluation of Environmental-Factors and Programs." *Health Education Quarterly* Supplement: 2. S107–S127.

Giger, J. N., and R. E. Davidhizar. 1995. *Transcultural Nursing Assessment and Intervention,* 2nd ed. St. Louis: Mosby-Year Book.

Green, L. W., and M. W. Kreuter. 1999. *Health Promotion Planning: An Educational and Ecological Approach.* MountainView, CA: Mayfield.

McKenzie, J. F., B. L. Neiger, and R. Thackeray. 2013. *Planning, Implementing, and Evaluating Health Promotion Programs: A Primer.* Boston: Pearson Education.

Peoples-Sheps MD, A. Farel, and M. M. Rogers. 1996. *Assessment of Health Status Problems.* Washington, DC: Maternal and Child Health Bureau.

Simons-Morton, B. G., W. H. Greene, and N. H. Gottlieb. 1995. *Introduction to Health Education and Health Promotion.* Prospect Heights, IL: Waveland.

Epilogue

You have just been introduced to health education and health promotion. You are now clear about what health is, its dimensions, and its determinants. Hopefully this has been a grand journey for you since you first met the Helpums. Perhaps you have learned how to help individuals, families, and communities to change behaviors that can damage their health. Perhaps you have learned how to help individuals gain greater balance in their lives with improved spiritual, physical, psychological, and social health.

As students of public health or community health, you are most likely further along in planning for a career in the health care field than you were when you began the book. Now, not only can you consider making populations at home or abroad healthier with improved opportunities to live healthier and happier lives, but you also know the basics for doing this through the health education process for program planning to provide those opportunities.

Let us visit with the Helpum family again. They are having another family reunion two years later than when we first met them. Now observe them and their health. Do you see any changes? Are there health enhancing changes?

Part II. The Helpum Family: A Picture of Health?

Grandma Helpum is so excited today, because her son and his family have travelled a long way and are visiting her today. Every two years, all of the Helpum family members try to come together at her home to reminisce and enjoy each other's company. She misses her family still, but she has been so busy with her work in the community garden and the seniors club. The health education specialist that she met two years ago encouraged her to participate in a community health project for seniors, and she loves it. She gets out of her house, meets new people, and builds really happy relationships. She is learning all that she can about gardening so that she can begin a club at her church too. She is feeling so happy and healthy, she has found energy that she never had before. She is just so excited to see her family and know how they are doing.

Grandma Helpum's daughter-in-law, Cheryl, is truly radiant today. Cheryl gave up one of her two jobs last year after she and her husband, Carl, sought financial counseling, and are making a real dent in their debt problems. Grandma thinks that Cheryl is actually looking younger. For some reason, Cheryl began Tai Chi training once she cut back on work. She felt so good that she began a walking project. She consulted the health education specialist at the health department about her eating behavior and stress relief. She is feeling great! She and Carl are experiencing a rebirth of romance in their marriage. Now, if she can just get him to slow down a little more at work.

Carl Helpum, Grandma Helpum's son, is looking good too! He is still working hard, because he loves his work now. He has stopped focusing on those who want his job and is going through a spiritual renewal program at church. The church began a heart health promotion program and asked the leaders in the church to participate first. He has been involved in a regular exercise program four days per week and he is eating much better and drinking a lot less alcohol. He is enjoying his life with his family. He and Cheryl spend more quality time together. He has even found more time to spend with their son Michael.

Michael has had a rough year. He was released from the county jail three months ago after serving 15 months on a drunk driving charge. He has to now rebuild his life; he lost his great job at the bank. Michael thinks that his arrest and jail sentence was a wake-up call. He thought that he was invincible. While in jail, he worked with the chaplain and the health education specialist to get his life on the right track and he worked hard to turn his life around. It is not easy, but his parents and sister have been very supportive. He takes one day at a time and avoids his old drug and drinking buddies. His new job is a starting position with a marketing firm. He participates in the worksite wellness program that offers nutrition and physical fitness training. These activities keep his mind off of the things that got him into trouble two years ago.

Trish loves her grandmother and is delighted to spend time with her. She is 20 years old now and has matured greatly. She has agreed to work part-time to pay for her college education. She is planning to move and live with Grandma Helpum when she graduates from college. She will look for employment in her grandmother's hometown. She is so grateful to her mother and grandmother for helping her turn her life around over the past two years. Two years ago, Trish thought that she was pregnant and was afraid to tell her parents, but Grandma Helpum suspected that something was wrong with Trish and her hesitancy to interact with her family during the last reunion. Grandma Helpum pulled her aside and encouraged Trish to share her concerns. Trish broke down crying and told them of her fear of being pregnant. This opened up lines of communication and guidance with Trish, her parents, and grandmother. When she returned to college she arranged for a pregnancy test. She was not pregnant. She was gaining more weight, probably because of the stress of relationships that were not at all fulfilling and causing her to eat as a stress reliever. Trish began attending the college's wellness center. She attended a number of sessions that covered sex education, nutrition education, physical fitness, and decision-making for college students. Trish is now focused on her future. If the right man comes along, she will know it and will wait for him rather than having so many unfulfilling interactions with men that she hardly knows. She is focused and really looking good and feeling good!

Here comes Grandma Helpum with her camera as always. "Let's take pictures! I want all of my friends to see my beautiful and healthy family!"

Application Opportunity

Activity A

1. You, the reader, are invited to look more closely at Grandma Helpum's photographs of her family two years ago and now. What do you see?

2. The Helpums are a fictional family, but do they provide a snapshot of the typical American way of living—and dying? Explain.

3. How did health education and health promotion impact each of their lives?

4. What would you say about the changes and health status of each family member now?

    *   Grandma Helpum

    *   Carl Helpum

    *   Cheryl Helpum

    *   Trish Helpum

    *   Michael Helpum

Activity B

As you observed the Helpums, perhaps you used your own definitions and standards for health, illness and disease in assessing this family.

1. Has your definition of health and disease changed since you began this textbook? How has it changed?

2. Are you now considering health education and health promotion as a career field? Why or why not?

3. How do you see health education and health promotion impacting the lives of individuals, families and communities locally, nationally, and globally?

Appendix A

Code of Ethics for the Health Education Profession Preamble

The Health Education profession is dedicated to excellence in the practice of promoting individual, family, group, organizational, and community health. Guided by common goals to improve the human condition, Health Educators are responsible for upholding the integrity and ethics of the profession as they face the daily challenges of making decisions. Health Educators value diversity in society and embrace a multiplicity of approaches in their work to support the worth, dignity, potential, and uniqueness of all people.

The Code of Ethics provides a framework of shared values within the professions in which Health Education is practiced. The Code of Ethics is grounded in fundamental ethical principles including: promoting justice, doing good, and avoidance of harm. The responsibility of each health educator is to aspire to the highest possible standards of conduct and to encourage the ethical behavior of all those with whom they work.

Regardless of job title, professional affiliation, work setting, or population served, Health Educators should promote and abide by these guidelines when making professional decisions.

Article I: Responsibility to the Public

A Health Educator's responsibilities are to educate, promote, maintain, and improve the health of individuals, families, groups and communities. When a conflict of issues arises among individuals, groups, organizations, agencies, or institutions, health educators must consider all issues and give priority to those that promote the health and well-being of individuals and the public while respecting both the principles of individual autonomy, human rights and equality.

Section 1: Health Educators support the right of individuals to make informed decisions regarding their health, as long as such decisions pose no risk to the health of others.

Section 2: Health Educators encourage actions and social policies that promote maximizing health benefits and eliminating or minimizing preventable risks and disparities for all affected parties.

Section 3: Health Educators accurately communicate the potential benefits, risks and/or consequences associated with the services and programs that they provide.

Section 4: Health Educators accept the responsibility to act on issues that can affect the health of individuals, families, groups and communities.

Section 5: Health Educators are truthful about their qualifications and the limitations of their education, expertise and experience in providing services consistent with their respective level of professional competence.

Section 6: Health Educators are ethically bound to respect, assure, and protect the privacy, confidentiality, and dignity of individuals.

Section 7: Health Educators actively involve individuals, groups, and communities in the entire educational process in an effort to maximize the understanding and personal responsibilities of those who may be affected.

Section 8: Health Educators respect and acknowledge the rights of others to hold diverse values, attitudes, and opinions.

Section 9: Health educators provide services equitably to all people.

Article II: Responsibility to the Profession

Health Educators are responsible for their professional behavior, for the reputation of their profession, and for promoting ethical conduct among their colleagues.

Section 1: Health Educators maintain, improve, and expand their professional competence through continued study and education; membership, participation, and leadership in professional organizations; and involvement in issues related to the health of the public.

Section 2: Health Educators model and encourage nondiscriminatory standards of behavior in their interactions with others.

Section 3: Health Educators encourage and accept responsible critical discourse to protect and enhance the profession.

Section 4: Health Educators contribute to the profession by refining existing and developing new practices, and by sharing the outcomes of their work.

Section 5: Health Educators are aware of real and perceived professional conflicts of interest, and promote transparency of conflicts.

Section 6: Health Educators give appropriate recognition to others for their professional contributions and achievements.

Section 7: Health educators openly communicate to colleagues, employers and professional organizations when they suspect unethical practice that violates the profession's Code of Ethics.

Article III: Responsibility to Employers

Health Educators recognize the boundaries of their professional competence and are accountable for their professional activities and actions.

Section 1: Health Educators accurately represent their qualifications and the qualifications of others whom they recommend.

Section 2: Health Educators use and apply current evidence-based standards, theories, and guidelines as criteria when carrying out their professional responsibilities.

Section 3: Health Educators accurately represent potential and actual service and program outcomes to employers.

Section 4: Health Educators anticipate and disclose competing commitments, conflicts of interest, and endorsement of products.

Section 5: Health Educators acknowledge and openly communicate to employers, expectations of job-related assignments that conflict with their professional ethics.

Section 6: Health Educators maintain competence in their areas of professional practice.

Section 7: Health Educators exercise fiduciary responsibility and transparency in allocating resources associated with their work.

Article IV: Responsibility in the Delivery of Health Education

Health Educators deliver health education with integrity. They respect the rights, dignity, confidentiality, and worth of all people by adapting strategies and methods to the needs of diverse populations and communities.

Section 1: Health Educators are sensitive to social and cultural diversity and are in accord with the law, when planning and implementing programs.

Section 2: Health Educators remain informed of the latest advances in health education theory, research, and practice.

Section 3: Health educators use strategies and methods that are grounded in and contribute to the development of professional standards, theories, guidelines, data and experience.

Section 4: Health Educators are committed to rigorous evaluation of both program effectiveness and the methods used to achieve results.

Section 5: Health Educators promote the adoption of healthy lifestyles through informed choice rather than by coercion or intimidation.

Section 6: Health Educators communicate the potential outcomes of proposed services, strategies, and pending decisions to all individuals who will be affected.

Section 7: Health educators actively collaborate and communicate with professionals of various educational backgrounds and acknowledge and respect the skills and contributions of such groups.

Article V: Responsibility in Research and Evaluation

Health Educators contribute to the health of the population and to the profession through research and evaluation activities. When planning and conducting research or evaluation, health educators do so in accordance with federal and state laws and regulations, organizational and institutional policies, and professional standards.

Section 1: Health Educators adhere to principles and practices of research and evaluation that do no harm to individuals, groups, society, or the environment.

Section 2: Health Educators ensure that participation in research is voluntary and is based upon the informed consent of the participants.

Section 3: Health Educators respect and protect the privacy, rights, and dignity of research participants, and honor commitments made to those participants.

Section 4: Health Educators treat all information obtained from participants as confidential unless otherwise required by law. Participants are fully informed of the disclosure procedures.

Section 5: Health Educators take credit, including authorship, only for work they have actually performed and give appropriate credit to the contributions of others.

Section 6: Health Educators who serve as research or evaluation consultants maintain confidentiality of results unless permission is granted or in order to protect the health and safety of others

Section 7: Health Educators report the results of their research and evaluation objectively, accurately, and in a timely fashion to effectively foster the translation of research into practice.

Section 8: Health Educators openly share conflicts of interest in the research, evaluation, and dissemination process.

Article VI: Responsibility in Professional Preparation

Those involved in the preparation and training of Health Educators have an obligation to accord learners the same respect and treatment given other groups by providing quality education that benefits the profession and the public.

Section 1: Health Educators select students for professional preparation programs based upon equal opportunity for all, and the individual's academic performance, abilities, and potential contribution to the profession and the public's health.

Section 2: Health Educators strive to make the educational environment and culture conducive to the health of all involved, and free from all forms of discrimination and harassment.

Section 3: Health Educators involved in professional preparation and development engage in careful planning; present material that is accurate, developmentally and culturally appropriate; provide reasonable and prompt feedback; state clear and reasonable expectations; and conduct fair assessments and prompt evaluations of learners.

Section 4: Health Educators provide objective, comprehensive, and accurate counseling to learners about career opportunities, development, and advancement, and assist learners in securing professional employment or further educational opportunities.

Section 5: Health Educators provide adequate supervision and meaningful opportunities for the professional development of learners.

Task Force Members:

Michael Ballard

Brian Colwell

Suzanne Crouch

Mal Goldsmith, Chairperson

Marc Hiller

Adrian Lyde

Lori Phillips

Catherine Rasberry

Raymond Rodriquez

Terry Wessel

Appendix B

Areas of Responsibilities, Competencies, and Sub-competencies for the Health Education Specialists 2010

The Seven Areas of Responsibility contain a comprehensive set of Competencies and Sub-competencies defining the role of the health education specialist. These Responsibilities were verified through the 2010 Health Educator Job Analysis Project and serve as the basis of the CHES exam beginning in April 2011 and the MCHES exam in October 2011. The Sub-competencies shaded are advanced-level only and will not be included in the entry-level, CHES examination. However the advanced-level Sub-competencies will be included in the October 2011 MCHES examination.

Area of Responsibility I:

Assess Needs, Assets, and Capacity for Health Education

COMPETENCY 1.1. Plan Assessment Process

1.1.1   Identify existing and needed resources to conduct assessments

1.1.2   Identify stakeholders to participate in the assessment process

1.1.3   Apply theories and models to develop assessment strategies

1.1.4   Develop plans for data collection, analysis, and interpretation

1.1.5   Engage stakeholders to participate in the assessment process

1.1.6   Integrate research designs, methods, and instruments into assessment plan

Reprinted by permission of The National Commission for Health Education Credentialing, Inc., Society for Public Health Education (SOPHE), and American Association for Health Education (AAHE).

COMPETENCY 1.2: Access Existing Information and Data Related to Health

1.2.1. Identify sources of data related to health

1.2.2. Critique sources of health information using theory and evidence from the literature

1.2.3. Select valid sources of information about health

1.2.4. Identify gaps in data using theories and assessment models

1.2.5. Establish collaborative relationships and agreements that facilitate access to data

1.2.6. Conduct searches of existing databases for specific health-related data

COMPETENCY 1.3: Collect Quantitative and/or Qualitative Data Related to Health

1.3.1. Collect primary and/or secondary data

1.3.2. Integrate primary data with secondary data

1.3.3. Identify data collection instruments and methods

1.3.4. Develop data collection instruments and methods

1.3.5. Train personnel and stakeholders regarding data collection

1.3.6 Use data collection instruments and methods

1.3.7 Employ ethical standards when collecting data

COMPETENCY 1.4: Examine Relationships Among Behavioral, Environmental, and Genetic Factors That Enhance or Compromise Health

1.4.1. Identify factors that influence health behaviors

1.4.2. Analyze factors that influence health behaviors

1.4.3. Identify factors that enhance or compromise health

1.4.4. Analyze factors that enhance or compromise health

COMPETENCY 1.5: Examine Factors That Influence the Learning Process

1.5.1. Identify factors that foster or hinder the learning process

1.5.2. Analyze factors that foster or hinder the learning process

1.5.3. Identify factors that foster or hinder attitudes and belief

1.5.4. Analyze factors that foster or hinder attitudes and beliefs

1.5.5 Identify factors that foster or hinder skill building

1.5.6 Analyze factors that foster or hinder skill building

Reprinted by permission of The National Commission for Health Education Credentialing, Inc., Society for Public Health Education (SOPHE), and American Association for Health Education (AAHE).

COMPETENCY 1.6: Examine Factors That Enhance or Compromise the Process of Health Education

1.6.1. Determine the extent of available health education programs, interventions, and policies

1.6.2. Assess the quality of available health education programs, interventions, and policies

1.6.3. Identify existing and potential partners for the provision of health education

1.6.4. Assess social, environmental, and political conditions that may impact health education

1.6.5. Analyze the capacity for developing needed health education

1.6.6. Assess the need for resources to foster health education

COMPETENCY 1.7: Infer Needs for Health Education Based on Assessment Findings

1.7.1. Analyze assessment findings

1.7.2. Synthesize assessment findings

1.7.3. Prioritize health education needs

1.7.4. Identify emerging health education needs

1.7.5. Report assessment findings

Area of Responsibility II:

Plan Health Education

COMPETENCY 2.1: Involve Priority Populations and Other Stakeholders in the Planning Process

2.1.1. Incorporate principles of community organization

2.1.2. Identify priority populations and other stakeholders

2.1.3. Communicate need for health education to priority populations and other stakeholders

2.1.4. Develop collaborative efforts among priority populations and other stakeholders

2.1.5. Elicit input from priority populations and other stakeholders

2.1.6. Obtain commitments from priority populations and other stakeholders

COMPETENCY 2.2: Develop Goals and Objectives

2.2.1   Use assessment results to inform the planning process

2.2.2   Identify desired outcomes utilizing the needs assessment results

2.2.3 Select planning model(s) for health education

2.2.4 Develop goal statements

2.2.5 Formulate specific, measurable, attainable, realistic, and time-sensitive objectives

2.2.6 Assess resources needed to achieve objectives

COMPETENCY 2.3: Select or Design Strategies and Interventions

2.3.1 Assess efficacy of various strategies to ensure consistency with objectives

2.3.2 Design theory-based strategies and interventions to achieve stated objectives

2.3.3 Select a variety of strategies and interventions to achieve stated objectives

2.3.4 Comply with legal and ethical principles in designing strategies and interventions

2.3.5 Apply principles of cultural competence in selecting and designing strategies and interventions

2.3.6 Pilot test strategies and interventions

COMPETENCY 2.4: Develop a Scope and Sequence for the Delivery of Health Education

2.4.1 Determine the range of health education needed to achieve goals and objectives

2.4.2 Select resources required to implement health education

2.4.3 Use logic models to guide the planning process

2.4.4 Organize health education into a logical sequence

2.4.5 Develop a timeline for the delivery of health education

2.4.6 Analyze the opportunity for integrating health education into other programs

2.4.7 Develop a process for integrating health education into other programs

COMPETENCY 2.5: Address Factors That Affect Implementation

2.5.1 Identify factors that foster or hinder implementation

2.5.2 Analyze factors that foster or hinder implementation

2.5.3 Use findings of pilot to refine implementation plans as needed

2.5.4 Develop a conducive learning environment

Area of Responsibility III:

Implement Health Education

COMPETENCY 3.1: Implement a Plan of Action

3.1.1   Assess readiness for implementation

3.1.2   Collect baseline data

3.1.3   Use strategies to ensure cultural competence in implementing health education plans

3.1.4   Use a variety of strategies to deliver a plan of action

3.1.5   Promote plan of action

3.1.6   Apply theories and models of implementation

3.1.7   Launch plan of action

COMPETENCY 3.2: Monitor Implementation of Health Education

3.2.1   Monitor progress in accordance with timeline

3.2.2   Assess progress in achieving objectives

3.2.3   Modify plan of action as needed

3.2.4   Monitor use of resources

3.2.5   Monitor compliance with legal and ethical principles

COMPETENCY 3.3: Train Individuals Involved in Implementation of Health Education

3.3.1   Select training participants needed for implementation

3.3.2   Identify training needs

3.3.3   Develop training objectives

3.3.4   Create training using best practices

3.3.5   Demonstrate a wide range of training strategies

3.3.6   Deliver training

3.3.7   Evaluate training

3.3.8   Use evaluation findings to plan future training

Area of Responsibility IV:

Conduct Evaluation and Research Related to Health Education

COMPETENCY 4.1: Develop Evaluation/Research Plan

4.1.1   Create purpose statement

4.1.2   Develop evaluation/research questions

Reprinted by permission of The National Commission for Health Education Credentialing, Inc., Society for Public Health Education (SOPHE), and American Association for Health Education (AAHE).

4.1.3   Assess feasibility of conducting evaluation/research

4.1.4   Critique evaluation and research methods and findings found in the related literature

4.1.5   Synthesize information found in the literature

4.1.6   Assess the merits and limitations of qualitative and quantitative data collection for evaluation

4.1.7   Assess the merits and limitations of qualitative and quantitative data collection for research

4.1.8   Identify existing data collection instruments

4.1.9   Critique existing data collection instruments for evaluation

4.1.10   Critique existing data collection instruments for research

4.1.11   Create a logic model to guide the evaluation process

4.1.12   Develop data analysis plan for evaluation

4.1.13   Develop data analysis plan for research

4.1.14   Apply ethical standards in developing the evaluation/ research plan

COMPETENCY 4.2: Design Instruments to Collect

4.2.1   Identify useable questions from existing instruments

4.2.2   Write new items to be used in data collection for evaluation

4.2.3   Write new items to be used in data collection for research

4.2.4   Establish validity of data collection instruments

4.2.5   Establish reliability of data collection instruments

COMPETENCY 4.3: Collect and Analyze Evaluation/Research Data

4.3.1   Collect data based on the evaluation/research plan

4.3.2   Monitor data collection and management

4.3.3   Analyze data using descriptive statistics

4.3.4   Analyze data using inferential and/or other advanced statistical methods

4.3.5   Analyze data using qualitative methods

4.3.6   Apply ethical standards in collecting and analyzing data

COMPETENCY 4.4: Interpret Results of the Evaluation/Research

4.4.1   Compare results to evaluation/research questions

4.4.2   Compare results to other findings

4.4.3   Propose possible explanations of findings

4.4.4   Identify possible limitations of findings

4.4.5   Develop recommendations based on results

Reprinted by permission of The National Commission for Health Education Credentialing, Inc., Society for Public Health Education (SOPHE), and American Association for Health Education (AAHE).

COMPETENCY 4.5: Apply Findings From Evaluation/Research

4.5.1   Communicate findings to stakeholders

4.5.2   Evaluate feasibility of implementing recommendations from evaluation

4.5.3   Apply evaluation findings in policy analysis and program development

4.5.4   Disseminate research findings through professional conference presentations

Area of Responsibility V:

Administer and Manage Health Education

COMPETENCY 5.1: Manage Fiscal Resources

5.1.1   Identify fiscal and other resources

5.1.2   Prepare requests/proposals to obtain fiscal resources

5.1.3   Develop budgets to support health education efforts

5.1.4   Manage program budgets

5.1.5   Prepare budget reports

5.1.6   Demonstrate ethical behavior in managing fiscal resources

COMPETENCY 5.2: Obtain Acceptance and Support for Programs

5.2.1   Use communication strategies to obtain program support

5.2.2   Facilitate cooperation among stakeholders responsible for health education

5.2.3   Prepare reports to obtain and/or maintain program support

5.2.4   Synthesize data for purposes of reporting

5.2.5   Provide support for individuals who deliver professional development opportunities

5.2.6   Explain how program goals align with organizational structure, mission, and goals

COMPETENCY 5.3: Demonstrate Leadership

5.3.1   Conduct strategic planning

5.3.2   Analyze an organization's culture in relationship to health education goals

5.3.3   Promote collaboration among stakeholders

5.3.4   Develop strategies to reinforce or change organizational culture to achieve health education goals

Reprinted by permission of The National Commission for Health Education Credentialing, Inc., Society for Public Health Education (SOPHE), and American Association for Health Education (AAHE).

5.3.5 Comply with existing laws and regulations

5.3.6 Adhere to ethical standards of the profession

5.3.7 Facilitate efforts to achieve organizational mission

5.3.8 Analyze the need for a systems approach to change

5.3.9 Facilitate needed changes to organizational cultures

COMPETENCY 5.4: Manage Human Resources

5.4.1 Develop volunteer opportunities

5.4.2 Demonstrate leadership skills in managing human resources

5.4.3 Apply human resource policies consistent with relevant laws and regulations

5.4.4 Evaluate qualifications of staff and volunteers needed for programs

5.4.5 Recruit volunteers and staff

5.4.6 Employ conflict resolution strategies

5.4.7 Apply appropriate methods for team development

5.4.8 Model professional practices and ethical behavior

5.4.9 Develop strategies to enhance staff and volunteers' career development

5.4.10 Implement strategies to enhance staff and volunteers' career development

5.4.11 Evaluate performance of staff and volunteers

COMPETENCY 5.5: Facilitate Partnerships in Support of Health Education

5.5.1 Identify potential partner(s)

5.5.2 Assess capacity of potential partner(s) to meet program goals

5.5.3 Facilitate partner relationship(s)

5.5.4 Elicit feedback from partner(s)

5.5.5 Evaluate feasibility of continuing partnership

Area of Responsibility VI:

Serve as a Health Education Resource Person

COMPETENCY 6.1: Obtain and Disseminate Health-Related Information

6.1.1 Assess information needs

6.1.2 Identify valid information resources

Reprinted by permission of The National Commission for Health Education Credentialing, Inc., Society for Public Health Education (SOPHE), and American Association for Health Education (AAHE).

6.1.3   Critique resource materials for accuracy, relevance, and timeliness

6.1.4   Convey health-related information to priority populations

6.1.5   Convey health-related information to key stakeholders

COMPETENCY 6.2: Provide Training

6.2.1.   Analyze requests for training

6.2.2   Prioritize requests for training

6.2.3   Identify priority populations

6.2.4   Assess needs for training

6.2.5   Identify existing resources that meet training needs

6.2.6   Use learning theory to develop or adapt training programs

6.2.7   Develop training plan

6.2.8   Implement training sessions and programs

6.2.9   Use a variety of resources and strategies

6.2.10   Evaluate impact of training programs

COMPETENCY 6.3: Serve as a Health Education Consultant

6.3.1   Assess needs for assistance

6.3.2   Prioritize requests for assistance

6.3.3   Define parameters of effective consultative relationships

6.3.4   Establish consultative relationships

6.3.5   Provide expert assistance

6.3.6   Facilitate collaborative efforts to achieve program goals

6.3.7   Evaluate the effectiveness of the expert assistance provided

6.3.8   Apply ethical principles in consultative relationships

Area of Responsibility VII:

Communicate and Advocate for Health and Health Education

COMPETENCY 7.1: Assess and Prioritize Health Information and Advocacy Needs

7.1.1   Identify current and emerging issues that may influence health and health education

7.1.2   Access accurate resources related to identified issues

7.1.3   Analyze the impact of existing and proposed policies on health

7.1.4   Analyze factors that influence decision-makers

COMPETENCY 7.2: Identify and Develop a Variety of Communication Strategies, Methods, and Techniques

7.2.1   Create messages using communication theories and models

7.2.2   Tailor messages to priority populations

7.2.3   Incorporate images to enhance messages

7.2.4   Select effective methods or channels for communicating to priority populations

7.2.5   Pilot test messages and delivery methods with priority populations

7.2.6   Revise messages based on pilot feedback.

COMPETENCY 7.3: Deliver Messages Using a Variety of Strategies, Methods, and Techniques

7.3.1   Use techniques that empower individuals and communities to improve their health

7.3.2   Employ technology to communicate to priority populations

7.3.3   Evaluate the delivery of communication strategies, methods, and techniques

COMPETENCY 7.4: Engage in Health Education Advocacy

7.4.1   Engage stakeholders in advocacy

7.4.2   Develop an advocacy plan in compliance with local, state, and/or federal policies and procedures

7.4.3   Comply with organizational policies related to participating in advocacy

7.4.4   Communicate the impact of health and health education on organizational and socio-ecological factors

7.4.5   Use data to support advocacy messages

7.4.6   Implement advocacy plans

7.4.7   Incorporate media and technology in advocacy

7.4.8   Participate in advocacy initiatives

7.4.9   Lead advocacy initiatives

7.4.10 Evaluate advocacy efforts

COMPETENCY 7.5: Influence Policy to Promote Health

7.5.1   Use evaluation and research findings in policy analysis

7.5.2   Identify the significance and implications of health policy for individuals, groups, and communities

7.5.3   Advocate for health-related policies, regulations, laws, or rules

7.5.4   Use evidence-based research to develop policies to promote health

7.5.5   Employ policy and media advocacy techniques to influence decision-makers

COMPETENCY 7.6: Promote the Health Education Profession

7.6.1   Develop a personal plan for professional growth and service

7.6.2   Describe state-of-the-art health education practice

7.6.3   Explain the major responsibilities of the health education specialist in the practice of health education

7.6.4   Explain the role of health education associations in advancing the profession

7.6.5   Explain the benefits of participating in professional organizations

7.6.6   Facilitate professional growth of self and others

7.6.7   Explain the history of the health education profession and its current and future implications for professional practice

7.6.8   Explain the role of credentialing in the promotion of the health education profession

7.6.9   Engage in professional development activities

7.6.10 Serve as a mentor to others

7.6.11 Develop materials that contribute to the professional literature

7.6.12 Engage in service to advance the health education profession

Reference

National Commission for Health Education Credentialing, Inc. (NCHEC), Society for Public Health Education (SOPHE), American Association for Health Education (AAHE). (2010a). *A competency-based framework for health education specialists–2010.* Whitehall, PA: Author.

Appendix C

American Association for Health Education 2008 NCATE Health Education Teacher Preparation Standards

Standard I:

Content Knowledge: Candidates demonstrate the knowledge and skills of a health literate educator.

Key Element A: Candidates describe the theoretical foundations of health behavior and principles of learning.
Key Element B: Candidates describe the National Health Education Standards.
Key Element C: Candidates describe practices that promote health or safety.
Key Element D: Candidates describe behaviors that might compromise health or safety.
Key Element E: Candidates describe disease etiology and prevention practices.
Key Element F: Candidates demonstrate the health literacy skills of an informed consumer of health products and services.

Standard II:

Needs Assessment: Candidates assess needs to determine priorities for school health education.

Key Element A: Candidates access a variety of reliable data sources related to health.
Key Element B: Candidates collect health-related data.
Key Element C: Candidates infer needs for health education from data obtained.

Standard III:

Planning: Candidates plan effective comprehensive school health education curricula and programs.

Key Element A: Candidates design strategies for involving key individuals and organizations in program planning for School Health Education.
Key Element B: Candidates design a logical scope and sequence of learning experiences that accommodate all students.
Key Element C: Candidates create appropriate and measure-able learner objectives that align with assessments and scoring guides.
Key Element D: Candidates select developmentally appropriate strategies to meet learning objectives.
Key Element E: Candidates align health education curricula with needs assessment data and the National Health Education Standards.
Key Element F: Candidates analyze the feasibility of implementing selected strategies.

Standard IV:

Implementation: Candidates implement health education instruction.

Key Element A: Candidates demonstrate multiple instructional strategies that reflect effective pedagogy, and health education theories and models that facilitate learning for all students.
Key Element B: Candidates utilize technology and resources that provide instruction in challenging, clear and compelling ways and engage diverse learners.
Key Element C: Candidates exhibit competence in classroom management.
Key Element D: Candidates reflect on their implementation practices, adjusting objectives, instructional strategies and assessments as necessary to enhance student learning.

Standard V:

Assessment: Candidates assess student learning.

Key Element A: Candidates develop assessment plans.
Key Element B: Candidates analyze available assessment instruments.
Key Element C: Candidates develop instruments to assess student learning.
Key Element D: Candidates implement plans to assess student learning.
Key Element E: Candidates utilize assessment results to guide future instruction.

Standard VI:
Administration and Coordination: Candidates plan and coordinate a school health education program.

Key Element A: Candidates develop a plan for comprehensive school health education (CSHE) within a coordinated school health program (CSHP).
Key Element B: Candidates explain how a health education program fits the culture of a school and contributes to the school's mission.
Key Element C: Candidates design a plan to collaborate with others such as school personnel, community health educators, and students' families in planning and implementing health education programs.

Standard VII:
Being a Resource: Candidates serve as a resource person in health education.

Key Element A: Candidates use health information resources.
Key Element B: Candidates respond to requests for health information.
Key Element C: Candidates select educational resource materials for dissemination.
Key Element D: Candidates describe ways to establish effective consultative relationships with others involved in Coordinated School Health Programs.

Standard VIII:
Communication and Advocacy: Candidates communicate and advocate for health and school health education.

Key Element A: Candidates analyze and respond to factors that impact current and future needs in comprehensive school health education.
Key Element B: Candidates apply a variety of communication methods and techniques.
Key Element C: Candidates advocate for school health education.
Key Element D: Candidates demonstrate professionalism.

Index